Oklahoma Notes

Clinical Sciences Review for Medical Licensure
Developed at
The University of Oklahoma College of Medicine

Ronald S. Krug, *Series Editor*

Suitable Reviews for:
United States Medical Licensing Examination
(USMLE), Step 2
Federation Licensing Examination (FLEX)

Oklahoma Notes

Pediatrics

Edited by
A. Eugene Osburn

With Contributions by
Jill E. Adler   Patrice A. Aston
Jefry L. Biehler   Peggy J. Hines   Nancy R. Inhofe
Diane Kittredge   Thomas A. Lera   Jane E. Puls
G. Edward Shissler   Elias S. Srouji   Kendall L. Stanford
John H. Stuemky   Roger Thompson   James W. Worley
Richard W. Wright

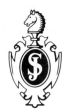

Springer-Verlag
New York Berlin Heidelberg London Paris
Tokyo Hong Kong Barcelona Budapest

Preface

One learns medicine, including pediatrics, by first learning a set of rules and then spending the rest of his/her productive career discovering exceptions to those rules. This book is intended to serve as a study guide for organizing the acquisition of an initial foundation of information about pediatric topics. Without an initial set of rules all new information is simply another new rule, and not an interpretive frame of reference for the deeper level of understanding that occurs with recognition that one is dealing with a change in his previously held belief. As such, I have attempted to include what I think most would agree are commonly held operational "facts" of pediatrics, and have not tried to justify or substantiate the facts with references or lengthy background information as to why these facts are currently thought to be true. My primary intent in writing this book is to provide an adequate core of pediatric information to enable one to pass the pediatric portion of the national boards. I hope it will also provide a foundation for those who wish to spend more time discovering why children are different. If this study guide fulfills whichever of these needs is yours, it will have been successful.

A. Eugene Osburn

Preface to the
Oklahoma Notes

In 1973 the University of Oklahoma College of Medicine instituted a requirement for passage of the Part 1 National Boards for promotion to the third year. To assist students in preparation for this examination a two-week review of the basic sciences was added to the Curriculum in 1975. Ten review texts were written by the faculty. In 1987 these basic science review texts were published as the *Oklahoma Notes* ("Okie Notes") and made available to all students of medicine who were preparing for comprehensive examinations. Over a quarter of a million of these texts have been sold nationally. Their clear, concise outline format has been found to be extremely useful by students preparing themselves for nationally standardized examinations.

Over the past few years numerous inquiries have been made regarding the availability of a Clinical Years series of "Okie Notes." Because of the obvious utility of the basic sciences books, faculty associated with the University of Oklahoma College of Medicine have developed texts in five specialty areas: Medicine, Neurology, Pediatrics, Psychiatry, and Surgery. Each of these texts follows the same condensed outline format as the basic science texts. The faculty who have prepared these texts are clinical educators and therefore the material incorporated in these texts has been validated in the classroom.

Each author has endeavored to distill the "need to know" material from their field of expertise. While preparing these texts, the target audience has always been the clinical years student who is preparing for Step 2 examinations.

A great deal of effort has gone into these texts. I hope they are helpful to you in studying for your licensure examinations.

Ronald S. Krug, Ph.D.
Series Editor

To Harriet, Greg, Hilary and my parents.

Oklahoma Notes

Pediatrics

Edited by
A. Eugene Osburn

With Contributions by
Jill E. Adler   Patrice A. Aston
Jefry L. Biehler   Peggy J. Hines   Nancy R. Inhofe
Diane Kittredge   Thomas A. Lera   Jane E. Puls
G. Edward Shissler   Elias S. Srouji   Kendall L. Stanford
John H. Stuemky   Roger Thompson   James W. Worley
Richard W. Wright

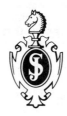

Springer-Verlag
New York Berlin Heidelberg London Paris
Tokyo Hong Kong Barcelona Budapest

A. Eugene Osburn, D.O.
Department of Pediatrics
College of Medicine
Health Sciences Center
The University of Oklahoma
Oklahoma City, OK 73190
USA

Library of Congress Cataloging-in-Publication Data
Pediatrics / edited by A. Eugene Osburn ; with contributions by Jill
  E. Adler . . . [et al.].
        p.   cm. — (Oklahoma notes)
    ISBN 0-387-97955-7 (pbk. : alk. paper) : $15.95. — ISBN
3-540-97955-7 (alk. paper)
    1. Pediatrics—Outlines, syllabi, etc.   I. Osburn, A. Eugene.
II. Series.
    [DNLM: 1. Pediatrics—outlines.   WS 18 P37025]
RJ48.3.P44   1992
618.92′0002′02—dc20
DNLM/DLC
for Library of Congress   92-49140
                                                        CIP

Printed on acid-free paper.

Production managed by Jim Harbison; manufacturing supervised by Jacqui Ashri.
Camera-ready copy prepared by the editor.
Printed and bound by Edwards Brothers, Inc., Ann Arbor, MI.
Printed in the United States of America.

9 8 7 6 5 4 3

ISBN 0-387-97955-7 Springer-Verlag New York Berlin Heidelberg
ISBN 3-540-97955-7 Springer-Verlag Berlin Heidelberg New York

Acknowledgments

I am grateful for the help and support provided by the secretaries, Phyllis Bullock, Jeannie Brown, Debby Williams, Tiffany Schoonover, and Christy Anthony in preparation of this manuscript. I especially appreciate the efforts of each of the contributors, who took time from their busy schedules to provide input from their areas of interest and expertise. Except as noted in the list of contributors, all are members of the Section of General Pediatrics, and all are especially accustomed to approaching the care of the child from a broad perspective. I am also grateful to Alfred W. Bann, Jr., M.D., Hobbs-Recknagel Professor and Chairman, Department of Pediatrics, and to John H. Stuemky, M.D., Chief, Section of General Pediatrics, Department of Pediatrics, and Medical Director, Ambulatory Care/Emergency Services, Children's Hospital of Oklahoma, for their encouragement and support in this endeavor. A special thank you is extended to James E. Wenzl, M.D., Professor and Vice Chairman for Clinical Affairs, Department of Pediatrics for his help with the study questions. The Editorial staff at Springer-Verlag was most helpful in providing assistance, guidance and encouragement. And finally, thank you to all the residents and students who asked me questions about topics in this book so many times that I finally got around to finding answers to some of them and writing them down. Each of the above individuals knows the significant portion of credit they deserve for this book. I want them to know I do too.

Contents

Contributors

Jill E. Adler, M.D.
Instructor
Department of Pediatrics
University of Oklahoma
College of Medicine
Oklahoma City, Oklahoma

Patrice A. Aston, D.O., FAAP
Private Practice, Oklahoma City
Clinical Assistant Professor
Department of Pediatrics
University of Oklahoma
College of Medicine
Oklahoma City, Oklahoma

Jefry L. Biehler, M.D.
Clinical Assistant Professor
Department of Pediatrics
University of Oklahoma
College of Medicine
Oklahoma City, Oklahoma

Peggy J. Hines, M.D., FAAP
Instructor
Department of Pediatrics
University of Oklahoma
College of Medicine
Oklahoma City, Oklahoma

Nancy R. Inhofe, M.D., FAAP
Assistant Professor
Department of Pediatrics
University of Oklahoma
College of Medicine;
Medical Director, Special
   Pediatric Clinic
Children's Hospital of Oklahoma
Oklahoma City, Oklahoma

Diane Kittredge, M.D., FAAP
Associate Professor
Department of Pediatrics
University of Oklahoma
College of Medicine;
Director, Pediatric Practice Model for
   Continuity Care
Children's Hospital of Oklahoma
Oklahoma City, Oklahoma

Thomas A. Lera, Jr., M.D., FAAP
Assistant Professor
Department of Pediatrics
University of Oklahoma
College of Medicine;
Associate Medical Director,
   Emergency Services;
Associate Chief of Staff
Children's Hospital of Oklahoma
Oklahoma City, Oklahoma

Jane E. Puls, M.D., FAAP
Assistant Professor
Former Director, Housestaff Education
Department of Pediatrics
University of Oklahoma
College of Medicine
Oklahoma City, Oklahoma

G. Edward Shissler, M.D., FAAP
Clinical Assistant Professor
Department of Pediatrics
University of Oklahoma
College of Medicine
Oklahoma City, Oklahoma

Elias S. Srouji, M.D., MPH, FAAP
Professor
Department of Pediatrics
University of Oklahoma
College of Medicine;
Former Medical Director, Diagnostic &
    Evaluation Clinic
Children's Hospital of Oklahoma
Oklahoma City, Oklahoma

Kendall L. Stanford, M.D., FAAP
Instructor
Director, House Staff Recruitment
Assistant Director, House
    Staff Education
Department of Pediatrics
University of Oklahoma
College of Medicine;
Associate Director,
Ambulatory Pediatric Clinic
Children's Hospital of Oklahoma
Oklahoma City, Oklahoma

John H. Stuemky, M.D., FAAP
Associate Professor
Chief, Section of General Pediatrics
Department of Pediatrics
University of Oklahoma
College of Medicine;
Medical Director, Ambulatory Care
    and Emergency Services
Children's Hospital of Oklahoma
Oklahoma City, Oklahoma

Roger Thompson, M.D.
Clinical Instructor
Department of Pediatrics
University of Oklahoma
College of Medicine
Oklahoma City, Oklahoma

James W. Worley, M.D., FAAP
Clinical Associate Professor
Department of Pediatrics
University of Oklahoma
College of Medicine
Oklahoma City, Oklahoma

Richard W. Wright, PhD
Professor
Biomedical Ethics and Research
Department of Pediatrics
Director, Biomedical and Health Care
Ethics Program for the
    Health Sciences Center
University of Oklahoma
College of Medicine
Oklahoma City, Oklahoma

Chapter 1 HEALTH MAINTENANCE CARE

Diane Kittredge
G. Edward Shissler
James Worley

The American Academy of Pediatrics Committee on Practice and Ambulatory Medicine provides guidelines for a systematic approach to Health Maintenance Care which includes the following components:

History
Physical Examination
Screening Procedures
      Growth curve measurements
            Height
            Weight
            Head Circumference
      Developmental Screening
      Cardiovascular Risk Screening
      Metabolic Screening
      Sensory Screening
      Hemoglobin/Hematocrit
      Urine dipstick
      Tuberculin test
      Lead screening
Immunizations
Anticipatory Guidance and Health Education

Health Maintenance Care visits are scheduled to evaluate the child in each of the above areas. Details of the age specific elements to be sought in each of these areas are found in numerous publications and practice protocols. The frequency of such visits is determined partially by the need to incorporate immunizations on a reasonable schedule, with additional visits scheduled to detect evolving problems as soon as practical. Listed in the tables below are highlights of such visits.

        The medical history and physical examination are guided by anticipated problems for the age being evaluated, as well by a Review of Systems and Complete Physical Exam to detect unanticipated problems.

Screening Procedures

Growth Screening

The height and weight should be plotted on age and sex appropriate growth curves at each visit. The head circumference should be measured and plotted for visits through age 18 months. Whether the child is following his/her curve is more important than any one individual measurement. Such growth curves are widely available. Below are methods for estimating expected growth parameters when such growth curves are not available.

The head circumference in term infants should grow at the following rate:

2 cm per month   for the 1st three months
1 cm per month   from 4-6 months
0.5 cm per month from 6-12 months

Height estimation

Height	Centimeters	Inches
At birth	50	20
At 1 year	75	30
2 - 12 years	age (yr) x 6 + 77	age (yr) x 2.5 + 30

Body weight estimation

Age	Weight (kg)	
Newborn	3.5	Birth Weight (BW)
6 months	7	2 x BW
1 year	10	3 x BW
4 years	17.5	1/4 AW
8 years	35	1/2 AW
adult	70	Adult Weight (AW)

Other growth parameters often useful to know are summarized in the following tables:

Surface area estimation guidelines

$$SA\ (M^2) = [A \times Weight] + B$$

Weight (kg)	A	B
0 to 5	0.05	0.05
6 to 10	0.04	0.10
11 to 20	0.03	0.20
21 to 40	0.02	0.40

The anterior fontanel should close to palpation by 18 months of age.
Causes of a larger than normal or persistently open fontanel are:

Athyrotic hypothyroidism	Alpert's syndrome
Malnutrition	Kenny's syndrome
Progeria	Aminopterin-induced syndrome
Rubella syndrome	Achondroplasia
Russell-Silver syndrome	Pyknodysostosis
Hallermann-Streiff syndrome	Vitamin D deficiency rickets
Down's syndrome	Osteogenesis imperfecta
Trisomy 13 syndrome	Hypophosphatasia
Trisomy 18 syndrome	Cleidocranial dysostosis

Expected age of deciduous teeth eruption

Tooth	Mean age (months)	Age range (months)
Lower central incisor	6	4-10
Upper central incisor	9	6-12
Upper lateral incisor	11.5	7-14
Lower lateral incisor	12	7-16
Upper first molar	15	12-18
Lower first molar	15.5	12-18
Lower cuspid	18	14-22
Upper cuspid	18	14-22
Lower second molar	26	22-30
Upper second molar	26	22-30

Developmental Screening

The child's developmental level should be assessed by history and examination at each visit. The Denver II is a widely used formal screening tool for ages 0 - 6 years. Below is a summary of highlights of developmental milestones for less formal use:

Age	Highlights of Developmental Milestones (Normal age range in months)	Developmental warning signs
2 weeks	Lifts chin when prone Lies in flexed position Fixates to close objects and light	Femoral click or hip instability (through 12 months) Undue maternal anxiety (true for months)
2 months	Smiles Squeals Follows objects with eyes past midline	Persistent heart murmur Absent response to noise Failure to fix gaze on face
4 months	Lifts head and chest from prone Smiles at others (1.5-4) Rolls over front to back Follows objects with eyes 180 degrees Grasps rattle Coos and says "ah"	Lack of bonding (a concern at any age)
6 months	Sits without support (5-8) Transfers objects hand to hand (4.5-7) Babbles	Failure to follow objects 180 degrees Persistent fisting Strabismus
9 months	Bears wieght Crawls Pincer grasp (8.5-12) Uncover hidden toy Says nonspecific "Mama-Dada" Cruises holding furniture	Nystagmus Absence of babble Unable to sit alone
12 months	Stands alone (10-14) Says "Mama " or" Dada" (9-13) Walks well (11-15) Tree words in addition to "Mama"	Unable to transfer objects hand to hand Absence of weight bearing while held
15 months	Walks backwards (12.5-21.5) Eats with a spoon	Unable to pull self to stand Abnormal grasp or pincer grip

18 months	Walks up steps (14-22) Finds hidden object (14-20) Stacks four cubes (15-20) Puts three words together	Open anterior fontanel Inability to walk alone Absence of constructive play Lack of spontaneous vocalization
24 months	Pedals tricycle (21-28) Combines 2 words (14-24) Kicks a ball forward on request	Absence of recognizable words
3 years	Uses plurals (21-36) Balances on one foot (30-44) Goes up stairs Knows age Counts three objects	Speech unintelligible to strangers
Preschool 3-6 years	Stands 10 seconds on one foot by 5 years By school age, knows colors, counts to 10 hops on one foot, can heel-toe walk and speaks sentences of at least 10 syllavles.	Inability to perform self care tasks: handwashing, simple dressing, daytime toilet
School age 6-12 years	Is able to take formal tests to assess developmental level of achievement Sexual maturation begins agound 10 years in girls and 12 years in boys	School failure Agressive behavior such as firesetting
Adolescence	Formal assessment tools can be used to quantitate level of functioning.	School absenteesm or school failure

Metabolic Screening

The newborn is screened for hypothyroidism and the hyperphenylalaninemias including phenylketonuria (PKU) after 24 hours of age to insure an adequate protein intake for valid results. Infants discharged early may require a repeat screening at 2 weeks of age. Other metabolic screening is dictated by family history and clinical suspicion. Some states routinely screen for a wide battery of metabolic disorders.

Sensory Screening

Hearing and vision are screened by subjective historical information and physical examination at each visit. Formal testing should be done before entering school, if not sooner because of a suspicious history or exam finding.

Hemoglobin/Hematocrit

Screen in late infancy (9-12 months), toddlers (24 months), once in the school years and least once after puberty.

Urinalysis

A urine dipstick for protein, blood and indications of infection (nitrate, leukocyte estrase) is recommended at least once in the preschool or school age period. Urinalysis and cultures are done if indicated by history or exam.

Tuberculin test

AAP and CDC recommend annual testing for children in high risk populations (exposed to higher rates of TB than the USA national average or at medical risk for TB). Routine testing for low risk groups is optional: at 12-15 months, school entry and once in adolescence.

Lead Screening

This requirement depends on the risk present where one lives.

Cardiovascular Risk Screening

Blood pressure is measured routinely for children > 3 years of age.
Blood lipid screening is done after 2 years of age if relevant family history and for all 18 year olds.

Childhood Immunizations

Table I is offered by both the AAP and ACIP as a means of integrating a resonable immunization schedule and a reasonable well child care schedule: Table II details acceptable variations in timing of routine immunizations. Schedules for starting immunizations late and other special circumstances can be found in the current AAP Redbook.

The number of inadequately immunized children is a national public health problem. If a child is seen for any reason other than significant acute illness, and is eligible for immunizations, such immunizations should be given.

TABLE I

Summary of Immunization Schedule

Schedule		Birth	2 Months	4 Months	6 Months	15-18 Months	4-6 Years	Every 10 years
Diphtheria	DPT		X	X	X	X	X	X
Tetanus			X	X	X	X	X	X TD
Pertussis			X	X	X	X	X	
Polio	OPV		X	X		X	X	
Measles	MMR					X	X	
Mumps						X	X	
Rubella						X	X	
Haemophilus Influenzae	HbCV		X	X	X *	X **		
Hepatitis B	HBV	X	X		X			

Depending on which Hib vaccine is used:
   * this dose may not be required
   ** this dose may be given at 12 months

TABLE II

AGE /INTERVAL STANDARDS FOR ROUTINE CHILDHOOD IMMUNIZATIONS
Adapted from AAP and ACIP

PRODUCT/DOSE	AGE OR INTERVAL RECOMMENDED
DPT	
Primary 1	Age 6-8 weeks
Primary 2	4 to 8 weeks after Primary 1
Primary 3	4 to 8 weeks after Primary 2
Primary 4	6 to 12 months after Primary 3
Booster	Before school entry
Trivalent Oral Polio	
Primary 1	Age 6 to 8 weeks
Primary 2	8 weeks after Primary 1
Primary 3	6 to 12 months after Primary 2 & after age 12 months
Booster	Before school entry
Inactivated Polio Vaccine	
Primary 1	Age 6 to 8 weeks
Primary 2	4 to 8 weeks after Primary 1
Primary 3	6 to 12 months after Primary 2
Booster	Before school entry
Hemophilus Influenzae Type b	
Primary 1	Age 6 to 8 weeks
Primary 2	8 weeks after Primary 1*
Primary 3	8 weeks after Primary 2**
Primary 4	Age 15 months***
Hepatitis B, HBsAg Positive Mother	
HBIG (Immune globulin)	At birth
Primary 1	At birth
Primary 2	Age 1 month
Primary 3	Age 6 months
Hepatitis B, HBsAg Negative Mother	
Primary 1	Birth to 8 weeks
Primary 2	8 weeks after Primary 1
Primary 3	Age 6 to 18 months, preferable at least 4 months after Primary 2

  * 8 week intervals preferred; use 4 week intervals if no opportunity to give later - for instance, family moving soon to underdeveloped country
 ** This dose not required if using PRP-OMP vaccine
*** Give this dose at 12 months of age if using PRP-OMP vaccine

Anticipatory Guidance

This includes counseling and advice given in the following areas:

Child development:
> Help parents understand and anticipate developmental milestones.
> Advise activities to optimize developmental progress.

Child behavior:
> Help parents understand and respond appropriately to normal stages of infant and child behaviors.
> Guide parent in psychosocial aspects of child rearing (e.g. child care, discipline)

Nutrition:
> Respond to concerns about feeding and mealtime behavior.
> Offer counseling to improve nutrition and establish healthy eatting habits for life.

Safety:
> Provide counseling about common injuries at each age period and recommend strategies to reduce risks.

Medical concerns:
> Anticipate potential risks for dysfunction and diseases, and provide counseling and health education as indicated. (e.g. flouride supplementation to reduce dental caries; anticipatory planning to provide optimal medical services for children with chronic diseases, etc.)

Leading Injury Deaths USA, Ages 0 - 14
1980-1985

Death rate/ 100,000/ year		Etiology	Prevention
8.1	# 1	Motor Vehicle Accident	
		Occupant:	Car seats < 4 years
			Seat belts > 4 years
		Pedestrian	Street safety
		and Bike	Helmets when biking,
		related:	skating, etc.
2.8	# 2	Drowning	Pool fences, life jackets, water safety and swimming lessons
2.3	# 3	House fires	Smoke alarms
1.9	# 4	Homicide	Child abuse prevention services, gun control, substance abuse services
0.7	# 5	Suffocation and strangulation	Product regulation: cribs, plastic bags, pacificers, toys, etc.
0.6	# 6	Unintentional firearms	guns unloaded and locked away

Common Safety Hazards by age group

Age range	Hazard	Prevention
Early Infancy	Crib Safety	Slats less than 2 3/8 inches apart
	Scald burns	Water-heater temperature < 120 F
	MVA injuries	Car seats
	Rolling off high surface	Do not leave unattended
	Foreign body aspiration	Keep small toys and objects out of reach
Late Infancy	Poisonous ingestions	Restrict access to poisonous substances
	Increased mobility	Protect from open windows, electric cords, wall sockets, stairways and water hazards
	MVA injuries	Forward facing car seat when > 20 lbs
Pre-school	Unsafe use of toys or perceived toys	Teach playground safety
		Do not allow access to guns, knifes, etc.
	Bites from "pets"	Teach appropriate respect for animals
	Auto/Pedestrian accidents	Teach traffic safety
School age	Bicycle accidents	Bicycle helmets
	Sports injuries	Protective equipment, supervised sports
	Drowning	Water Safety
Adolescence	Feelings of invulnerability	Education and support to lessen self and peer pressure induced vehicular, substance abuse, and sexually transmitted injuries.

11

John H. Stuemky

Fetal Growth and Developmental

Normal Gestation Period - 40 weeks (280 days from first day of LMP)
Preterm Gestation - Birth at less than 38 weeks gestation
Term Gestation - Birth at 38 to 42 weeks gestation
Post-term Gestation - Birth after 42 weeks gestation

Neonatal Period - First 28 days of life.

Gestational Age

In utero, the fetus develops primarily by cell hyperplasia (increase in number of cells) in the first half of normal gestation. It develops primarily by hypertrophy (increase in cell size) in the last trimester. Interference with somatic growth in the first part of fetal life will thus generally cause a overall symetrical growth retardation since the number of cells present, not the size of cells will be most affected. Inhibition of cell growth occurs primarily in conditions that prevent adequate nutrition of the cells in the last trimester. Infants so affected by malnutrition usually have disportionately large heads compared to their body size because the brain continues to grow whereas the body cells do not hypertrophy.

For prognostic and predictive value in knowing what to expect for the infant, it is useful to deduce the gestational age of the infant and compare that with the expected weight range for it's age. This allows classification of the infant as Small, Appropriate or Large for Gestational Age.

Small for gestational age

SGA babies had interference with either cell hyperplasia or hypertrophy. Although these infants are small, their cells may be able to function at a much more mature level than would be expected by their weight alone. This is especially noticeable in their ability to escape developing respiratory distress because their lungs are much more mature than their weight alone suggests.

Appropriate for gestational age

AGA babies grew within expected ranges for their gestational age.

Large for gestational age

LGA babies have a weight greater than the 90th percentile for their age. These infants have large cells, but the cell function may be markedly immature. They are especially prone to hypoglycemia problems. Infants of Diabetic Mothers, infants with Hyprops fetalis, and infants with Beckwith-Wiedemann syndrome are the most common causes of LGA babies.

Expected Growth Rate of the fetus and neonate	
Age	Rate
14 to 15 weeks	5g/day
20 weeks	10g/day
32 to 34 weeks	30g/day
First week postnatal	5% weight loss
Neonates after 1 week	20 - 30 gm/day

Formula Compositions

20 Kcal/oz - Meets nutritional, fluid, and electrolytes needs of term infants

24 Kcal/oz - Useful for preterm infants who cannot tolerate the volume load of regular formula.

Iron supplementation - Required by all infants

Vitamin supplementation - Vitamins A, D, C for breast fed infants

Fluid and electrolyte requirements:

water 100cc/kg/day

sodium 1 to 3 mEq/kg/day

potassium 1 to 2 mEq/kg/day

chloride 1 to 3 mEq/kg/day

Caloric requirements:

Term infants require 100-120 kCal/kg/day

Major Fetal Circulatory Transition Changes

Before birth, only 10-15 % of the fetal circulation perfuses the lungs. After transition to extrauterine life, the pulmonary blood is increased by 8-10 fold due to closure of the foramen ovale and ductus arteriosus. Before birth, oxygenated blood from the placenta flows to the right atrium from the inferior vena cava, and then to both ventricles because of an open foramen ovale. The left ventricle perfuses primarily the brain and myocardium and the right ventricle perfuses the aorta and lower body through an open ductus arteriosus before birth. After birth, blood flow is from the right atrium to the right ventricle and then through the lungs via the pulmonary artery, where it is oxygenated. The oxygenated blood is returned to the left atrium and ventricle for distribution to the systemic circulation via the aorta. Systemic venous return is back to the vena cava and hence to the right atrium. The direction of flow of blood through the ductus arteriosus changes after birth from the fetal direction of right to left to a left to right direction because of the relative increase in left-sided pressures in the circulatory system after birth. This left to right flow continues until the functional closure of the ductus at around 12 hours of age.

Delivery room management

The need for resuscitation is assessed by use of the APGAR score. It is routinely done at 1 minute and 5 minutes after birth.

APGAR SCORE			
Score:	0	1	2
Appearance	blue, pale	body pink, acrocyanosis	no cyanosis
Pulse	absent	< 100/minute	> 100/minute
Grimace	no response	grimace	sneeze or cough
Activity	flaccid	weak flexion	strong flexion
Respiratory effort	absent	weak, irregular	strong, regular

The infant is dried and provided necessary temperature support.

The eyes are protected from gonococcal ophthalmia with Silver nitrate or erythromycin ophthalmic ointment.

The infant is given intramuscular vitamin K to facilitate synthesis of coagulation factors.

A heel stick is done to measure the blood glucose level. A level below 30-40 mg/dl in the normal term infant is considered hypoglycemia for the first couple hours after birth. Thereafter, a level below 40 mg/dl is abnormal.

As soon as is feasible, the infant is presented to the mother to initiate infant-maternal bonding.

Identification of risk factors or problems dictate additional measures, as appropriate.

Intrapartum Insult Anticipation

Problems in the delivery room can be anticipated in the following high-risk pregnancies:
   Maternal diabetes of current illness
   Preterm or post term gestation (< 38 weeks or > 42 weeks)
   Fetal distress evidenced by fetal monitoring or meconuim staining
   Multiple gestations
   Preeclampsia
   Maternal antibiody sensitization from Rh or ABO incompatabilities
   Maternal vaginal bleeding from placenta abruption or previa
   Prolonged rupture of membranes

Common Birth Injuries

Injury	Intervention	Prognosis
Fractured clavicle	Imobilize arm 7-10 days	Complete healing in 4-6 weeks
Skull fracture	Rule depression	Usually asymptomatic, unless depressed
Bruises/ecchymosis	Monitor bilirubin	Can cause hyperbilirubinemia with readsorption
Cephalohematoma (subperiosteal: do not cross suture lines)	Monitor bilirubin and Hgb	resorbed in 2-3 months
Caput Succedaneum (edema crosses suture lines)	None needed	Resolve without sequelae
Facial paralysis		Resolve in 1-6 months, if periphreal nerve.
Brachial plexus Injury	Physical therapy	Most resolve in 3-6 months
Phrenic nerve paralysis		Most recover in 2-3 months

Respiratory Distress in the Newborn

Neonatal respiratory distress is one of the most common problems encountered in the newborn infant. Although the manifestations are those of the respiratory system, the causes may be due to any of the conditions listed in the following table. Signs of respiratory distress include: sustained respiratory rate over 60/minute, expiratory grunting, intercostal and sternal retractions, cyanosis, nasal flaring, or persistent cough.

Causes of Neonatal Respiratory Distress

Pulmonary Disorders
    Upper Airway Obstruction
    Coanal atresia
    Vocal cord paralysis
    Meconium aspiration
    Transient tachypnea of the newborn
    Pneumonia
    Hyline Membrane Disease
    Pneumothorax
    Pleural effusions
    Lung structural abnormalities
Cardiac Disorders
    Left-sided outflow obstruction
        Hypoplastic left heart
        Aortic Stenosis
        Coarctation of the aorta
    Cyanotic Heart disease
        Transposition of the great vessels

Total anomalous pulmonary venous return
Tricuspid atresia
Hypoplastic right heart
Right-sided outflow obstruction

Other Disorders
Hypothermia
Hyperthermia
Hypoglycemia
Polycythemia
Metabolic acidosis
CNS lesions
Neuromuscular lesions
Phrenic nerve palsy
Skeletal abnormalities

Neonatal Jaundice

Jaundice on the first day of life is always pathologic.

Physiologic Jaundice of the Newborn should meet the following criteria:

Jaundice is not present on day 1 after birth
The total bilirubin rises by less than 5 mg/dl/day
The bilirubin peaks by day 3-4 in term infants (day 5-7 in preterm infants)
The total bilirubin does not exceed 13 mg.dl in term infants (15 mg/dl in preterm)
The jaundice should not last more than one week in the term infant or 2 weeks in the preterm infant.

Jaundice which fails to meet the above criteria requires additional investigation.

Causes of unconjugated hyperbilirubinemia in the neonate

Increased Bilirubin Production
Increased hemolysis (increased reticulocyte count)
Coombs positive patients
Rh incompatability
ABO incompatability
Minor blood group sensitizations
Coombs negative patients
RBC structural defects
Spherocytosis
Elliptocytosis
Pyknocytosis

Stomacytosis
RBC enzyme defects
   Glucose 6-phosphate dehydrogenase deficiency
   Pyruviate kinase deficiency
   Hexokinase deficiency
Nonhemolytic bilirubin production
   Extravascular hemorrhage readsorption
   Polycythemia
   Entrohepatic recirculation

Decreased rate of conjugation of bilirubin
   Physiologic jaundice
   Crigler-Najjar syndrome
   Breast milk jaundice
   glucuronyl transferase deficiency, type II

Abnormalities of Bilirubin Excretion or Reabsorption
   Hepatitis
   Biliary atresia
   choledochal cyst
   Sepsis
   Metabolic disorders
      Glactosemia
      glycogen storage diseases
      cystic fibrosis
      hypothyroidism
   Bile duct obstruction

Conjugated hyperbilirubinemia in the neonate

Unconjugated hyperbilirubinemia in the neonate can usually be treated by phototherapy or exchange transfusion. Unconjugated hyperbilirubinemia is not responsive to such treatment. Its presence indicates a significant underlying injury to hepatic cells or cholestasis.

Kernicterus is the result of depostition of unconjugated bilirubin in brain cells. It rarely occurs in term infants at bilirubin levels below 20 mg/dl, although events such as sepsis, asphyxia, and prematurity can allow unconjugated bilirubin to cross the blood-brain barrier at much lower levels. Premature infants weighing less than 1000 g have developed kernicterus at levels of less than 10 mg/dl. Drugs that displace bilirubin from its binding sites on albumin also place infants at risk for kernicterus at lower levels.

Peggy Hines

Adolescents are not a homogenous group.

"Adolesence" is a period of life beginning with puberty and terminating with cessation of somatic growth. It is also a biopsychosocial process that may begin before puberty and extend well beyond the end of somatic growth, in which case it is culturally defined.

Developmental Considerations

Physical Development

Puberty is the period during which secondary sex characteristics begin to develop.

Hypothalamic-piturary changes:
Nocturnal sleep-related augmentation of pulsatile LH secretion secondary to an increase in pulsatile GnRH release

Decrease in hypothalamic and pituitary sensitivity to estradiol and testosterone

Increase in LH and FSH

In females, the development of a positive ovulation feedback system:
estrogen --> increase GnRH --> LH --> ovulation

Adrenal gland changes:
Increased secretiion of sex hormones. However these are not necessary for development of secondary sex characteristics.

Other pubertal changes:
Increased insulin secretion
Increased plasma somatomedic-C
Increased GHRH

Pubertal Development Highlights

Female	Male
Starts at age 8 - 13 years	Starts at age 9.5 - 13.5 years
Duration: 3 - 4 years	Duration: about 3 years
Breast development typically precedes pubic hair development	Testicular enlargement is the first change
Adult height reached in: mid-puberty	Adult height reached in: latter half of puberty

Sexual Maturation Stages (Tanner Staging)

FEMALE BREAST DEVELOPMENT

Stage I :   No glandular tissue, areola conforms to the chest line

Stage II :   Breast bud forms, areola widens and elevates

Stage III: Continued enlargement of breast bud; further elevation and enlargement of the areola; no separation of breast contours

Stage IV: Areola and papilla form a mound projecting from the breast contour

Stage V :   Breast adult size (variable); areola and breast in same plane with papilla (nipple) projecting above areola

PUBIC HAIR DEVELOPMENT (male and female)

Stage I :   No pubic hair

Stage II :   Small amount of long, slightly pigmented hair along base of scrotum and penis in the male or the labia majora in females

Stage III: Moderate amount of more curly, pigmented and coarser hair. Begins to spread laterally and over mons pubis

Stage IV: Resembles adult hair in coarseness and curliness. Does not extemd over medial surface of thighs

Stage V :   Adult type and quantity extending to medial thigh and in 80% of males along the linea alba

MALE GENITALIA DEVELOPMENT

Stage I :   Prepubertal, testes less than 1.5cc in volume

Stage II :   Testes enlarge, scrotal skin is thinner and reddish and scrotum is larger

Stage III: Testes and scrotum continue to grow. Length of penis increases

Stage IV: Testes and scrotum continue to grow, scrotum darkens, penis grows in width and length. The glans develops.

Stage V :   Testes, scrotum and penis are adult in size and shape.

OTHER PHYSICAL PUBERTAL CHANGES

Height Growth: Pubertal growth accounts for 20-25% of final adult height
Growth spurt is highly variable
Average growth spurt lasts 24-36 months

Weight Growth: Pubertal weight gain accounts for 50% of an individual's ideal adult body weight

Male/Female Differences:
Peak height velocity occurs about 18-24 months earlier in the female.
Peak height velocity in females averages 2 cm/year less than in the male.
Peak weight and height velocities coincide in males.

Psychosocial Developmental in Adolescents

Tasks of Adolescence:

1. Achieving independence from parents.
2. Adopting peer codes and life-styles.
3. Assigning increased importance to body image and accepting one's body image.
4. Establishing sexual, ego, vocational and moral identities.

Task	Early Adolescence	Mid-Adolescence	Late Adolesence
Independence	Less interest in parental activities	Conflict with parents peaks	Reacceptance of parents values
Body Image	Preoccupation with self and pubertal changes	General acceptance of body	Acceptance of pubertal changes
Peers	Intense relationships with same-sex friends Conformity to peer group values	Peak peer group involvement More time spent in sharing intimate relationships	Peer group less important Increased sexual activity and experimentation
Identity	Increase ability to reason abstractly Increased need for privacy Idealistic Test authority	Increased scope of feelings Increased creative & intellectual activities Feelings of omnipotence and immortality	Rational and realistic conscience Sense of perspective Ability to delay, set limits Practical vocational goals Refinement of moral, religious and sexual values

Legal issues of Adolescence in the United States

Mature minor are individuals aged 15 years or older who understand risks and benefits of services provided.

Emancipated minors are individuals aged 16 years and older who are married, joined the armed services, or are living on their own and are managing their own financial affairs.

State Laws vary in rights of adolescencents to receive care without parental consent. Most allow mature minors to obtain treatment for drug abuse, sexually transmitted diseases and pregnancy related issues without patental consent.

Confidentially is a central part of adolescent care. It may be breached when life is at risk.

Screening Measures

History: Open-ended approach, questionaires, look for hidden agenda
HEADSS interview (Home, Education, Activities, Drugs, Sex, Suicide)

Physical: Height, weight, blood pressure, vision and hearing testing
Skin: acne, facial hair
Eyes: myopia
Dentition: Dental caries, third set of molars
Neck: Thyroid, adenopathy
Breast: Development, masses, gynecomastia
Heart Sounds: Murmurs, clicks
Musculoskeletal: Scoliosis
Genitalia:
> Male: Stage of development, urethral discharge, scrotal or testicular masses. Inguinal hernia or adenopathy.
> Female: Stage of development, Pelvic exam yearly for all sexually active adolescents and as indicated.

Laboratory tests: Hgb/Hct -- look for anemia in adolescent females secondary to menses and poor diet.
Urine analysis: check for asymptomatic proteinuria, hematuria, glucosuria
Rubella titer: in females prior to becoming pregnant
PPD
Cholesterol: draw level in all at risk individuals based on family history.

<u>In sexually active teenagers</u>
> Females: annual Pap smear, cervical gonorrhea culture and chlamydia screening, syphilis serology, vaginal wet mount, pregnancy testing as indicated.
> Males: annual syphilis serology, urethral cultures for gonorrhea, chlamydia screening.
> Homosexual males: annual syphilis serology, urethral, rectal, and pharyngeal gonorrhea cultures chlamydia and hepatitis B screening, HIV testing.

Menstrual Disorders

Amenorrhea

Primary amenorrhea: no episodes of spontaneous uterine bleeding by 14-16 years of age with absent secondary sexual characteristics; or by 16-18 years of age regardless of normal secondary sexual characteristics.

Secondary amenorrhea: After previous uterine bleeding, no subsequent menses for 6 months or length of time equal to 3 previous cycles.

Evaluation of amenorrhea

Primary amenorrhea

Primary amenorrhea evaluation is directed toward determination of pubertal maturation and the presence or absence of internal genitalia. A bimanual pelvic or ultrasound, if necessary, should be done to establish the presence or absence of a uterus and ovaries. The results can then be used to focus on a cause of the amenorrhea as depicted in the following:

	UTERUS ABSENT	**UTERUS PRESENT**
BREAST ABSENT	Conclusion: genetic males; gonads produce Mullerian inhibiting factor but do not produce enough testosterone to induce normal male internal and external genitalia Karyotype (XY) Gonadal enzyme deficiency Agonadism (testicular regression)	Conclusion: lack of ovarian estrogen production. Mullerian system developed normally Folicle Stimulating hormone low: Hypogonadotropic hypogonadism Lesions of the CNS Kallman syndrome Pituitary gonadotropic deficiencies (chronic disease, anorexia nervosa) Folicle Stimulating hormone high: Gonadal dysgenesis 45,XO (Turner syndorme) Other X chomosome variants Pure XX or XY dysgenesis Gonadal enzyme deficiency
BREAST PRESENT	Conclusion: Testosterone/Karyotype: Female (XX) Mullerian agenesis Male (XY) Androgen insensitivity (testicular feminization)	Conclusion: Normal phenotypic female with normal Mullerian and pubertal development. Absent menses is due to outlet obstruction or lack of endometrial development and shedding. Cyclic pain present: Rule out vaginal obstruction imperforate hymen transverse vaginal septum Cyclic pain absent: Hypothalmic-pituitary-ovarian axis disturbance (evaluate as secondary amonorrhea)

Secondary amenorrhea

Always consider pregnancy as a cause even if the history given does not suggest the diagnosis. Once pregnancy has been ruled out, the evaluation focuses on the hypothalamic-pituitary-ovarian axis.

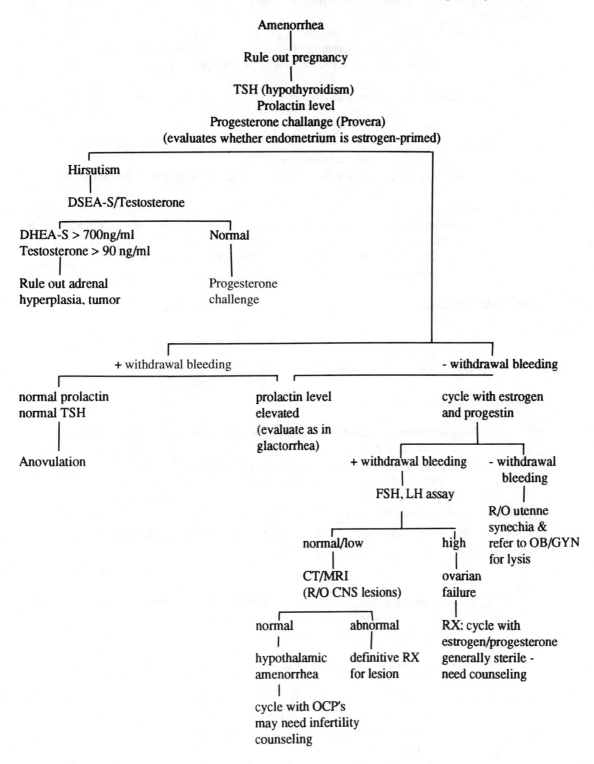

Dysmenorrhea:

> painful menstruation
> Most common gynecologic problem in adolescence
> occurs in 75% of menstruating women.

Etiology:
> Primagy Dysmenorrhea: No identifiable pelvic pathology.
>> Symptoms can be explained by the action of uterine prostaglandins
>>> (PGF2 alpha, PGE2 alpha, and cyclic endoperoxidases)

> Secondary dysmenorrhea: pain from endometriosis, infection or uterine fibroids.

Evaluation:
> History:
>> timing, character, and location of pain
>> past history of pelvic infection, intermenstrual bleeding, last menstrual period

> Pelvic Exam:
>> abnormal uterine position or shape suggest a uterine malformation (fibroids rare in adolescents)
>> cervical cultrues (chronic pelvic inflammatory disease may present as dysmenorrhea)

Differential diagnosis:
> Endometriosis
> PID
> Benign uterine tumors
> Anatomic abnormalities of the uterus

Treatment of primary dysmenorrhea:

> Oral Contraceptivces (reduce growth of endometrium and therefore decrease uterine prostaglandin production)
> Prostaglandin Inhibitors (block production of prostaglandins)
>> Mefanamic acid, naproxen, ibuprofen

Dysfunctional uterine bleeding

Abnormal endometial bleeding in the absence of structural pelvic pathology, usually associated with anovulation.

Pathophysiology:
> Estrogen stimulation of endometrium by corpus luteal progesterone causing overgrowth of the endometrium with patchy desquamation and sloughing.

Evaluation:
> **Immediate goals -- assess hemodynamic stability and identify site of bleeding.**

> History:
>> Bleeding disorder in patient or family?
>> History of easy bruising, epistaxis, gums bleeding?
>> Contraceptive use, IUD?
>> Sexual history, possibility of pregnancy?

Physical exam:
    Vital signs (orthostatic evaluation)
    Pelvic exam:
        evidence of trauma
        vaginal foreigh body
        ovarian masses
        signs of PID
        signs of pregnancy

Laboratory:
    CBC
    pregnancy test
    wet prep of vaginal discharge
    cervical cultures for gonorrhea, chlamydia
    thyroid studies, LFT's, clotting studies as indicated

Differential Diagnosis:
    Complications of pregnancy (ectopic, abortion, placental polyp)
    Endometritis
    Malignancy
    Cervical lesion
    Vaginal pathology (infection, polyp, foreign body, trauma)
    Ovarian dysfunction (polycystic ovarian syndrome, infection, tumors)
    Systemic disease (blood dyscrasias, cirrhosis, endocrine disorders)
    Iatrogenic (OPC's, tranquilizers, IUD)

Management: (based on severity of bleeding)

Mild: Inconvenient, unpredictable bleeding; hematocrit normal

    Consider oral contraceptive
    Reassurance
    Menstrual calendar
    Reevaluate in 3-6 months

Moderate: Irregular, prolonged, heavy bleeding; mild anemia (Hgb > 10g/dl)

    Hormonal therapy
        Medroxyprogesterone acetate OR oral contraceptives
    Iron supplementation
    Menstrual calendar
    Reevaluate every 1-3 months

Severe: Irregular, prolonged, heavy bleeding; moderate anemia (Hgb < 10g/dl)

    Not actively bleeding:
        Iron supplementation
        Oral contraceptive
        Reassurance
        Reevaluate every 1-3 months
    Actively bleeding:
        Hospitalize
        transfuse if indicated

Hormonal therapy
Conjugated estrogens IV q 4 hours X 6, concurrent
norgestrel/ethinynl estradiol 1 tablet q 6 hours to be
followed by OCP for 6-12 months
OR
Norgestrel/ethinyl estradiol 1 tablet q 6 hours for 24-48 hours
followed by OCP's for 6-12 months.
Dilatation and curettage if hormonal therapy fails
Reevaluate every month

Breast disorders

Asymmetry
Initial breast development may be asymmetric.
Asymmetry may be due to congenital absence of breast tissue.
Associated defects: absence of pectoral muscles or rib defects.
Treatment: Surgical treatment after puberty is finished to allow for full development
and equalization.

Accessory breast tissue
Most common breast anomaly.
Occurs in 1-2% of females.
Usually located on milk line, most commonly below breast on chest or upper abdomen.

Breast masses
Most masses found in adolescence are benign

Fibroadenoma
Benign neoplasm of mammary gland.
Most common breast lesion in middle and early female adolescents (76 - 90%
of benign lesions).

Physical Findings:
Firm, smooth, discrete mobile mass, lateral portion of breast commonly.
Usually less that 5 cm. in diameter.
Bilateral in 10 - 50%, multiple in 10%.

Fibrocystic Disease
Proliferation of stromal and epithelial elements of breast tissue with ductal
dilatation and cyst formation following in many individuals.

Pathophysiologic abnormality: Fibrocystic changes induced by excess
estrogen in relation to progesterone. Some studies implicate
Methylxanthines.

Symptoms: Tenderness, increased in late menstrual cycle.

Physical Findings: Cysts usually small, bilateral, firm, mobile. Nodularity -
hard and tender areas, 1 - 2 mm. to 1 cm in size.

Potential complications: Risk of breast cancer is increased five times in adult females who have proliferated fibrocystic lesions with atypia.

Management of Breast Lesions in Adolescents

Reassure adolescent that lesion is most likely benign. If breast mass feels cystic, aspiration can be done. Surgical removal of solid masses greater than 2-3 cm. in diameter. Observe most masses for at least 2 - 3 months before intervention -- resolution may occur following menstrual cycle. Mammography is not helpful in most cases. Never biopsy or excise a possible breast bud.

Gynecomastia

Excessive development of male mammary glands.

Etiology: Unknown, possibly an increase in biologically active estrogen or increased sensitivity to estrogen. Peak prevalence of 64% at age 14 years.

Pathology: Either 1) ductal proliferation and lobular formation or 2) stromal changes with fibrosis.

Symptoms: Tenderness on palption in some.

Physical Findings: Type I -- One or more subareolar nodules, freely mobile
Type II -- Breast nodules beneath the areola and extending beyond the areolar perimeter.
Type III -- Resenbkes breast development of sexual maturity stage 3 in female.
Also look for: Findings suggestive of hypogondism, hyper or hypothyroidism.
Testicular mass or atrophy.
Findings suggestive of liver disease.

Differential Diagnosis:
Drug exposure (estrogen, testosterone, phenothiazines, digoxin, tricyclics, phenytoin)
Renal failure.
Recovery from malnutrition.
Hypergonadotropic hypogonadism -- Klinefelter's syndrome.
Hyper- or hypothyroidism.
Tumors (testicular, bronchogenic, pituitary, adrenal, Hodgkins, hepatomas)
Liver disease.
Pseudogynecomastia (secondary to adipose in obese males or increased muscle tissue in the athletic).

Diagnostic Plan: In healthy pubertal males with normal growth no test are indicated. If gynecomastia occurs before the onset or after the completion of puberty, consider:
Karyotype
HCG level -- may be increase in various carcinomas
Serum estradiol -- feminizing adrenal tumors
Prolactin level, skull films -- pituitary tumors
Thyroid or liver function tests
Chest x-ray -- pulmonary tumors

Therapeutic Plan: Rule out other causes as above --
Reassurance and explanation
Consider surgery for massive gynecomastia or if it causes severe psychological problems.

Galactorrhea
Abnormal milky or watery discharge from one or both breasts in a nonpuerperal breast. Microscopic examination of discharge demonstrates fat goblets.

Etiology: Distruption of hypothalamic-pituitary control of prolactin secretion.

Differential Diagnosis: Drug use 1) tranquilizers, reserpine, methyldopa, opiates -- lead to decreased dopamine secretion. Dopamine inhibits prolactin secretion. 2) oral contraceptives -- secondary to LH and FSH suppression and increase in baseline prolactin.

Hypothyroidism -- elevated TRH increases prolactin secretion.

Pituitary Causes -- Adenomas (micro < 10 mm., macro > 10 mm.)
Empty sella syndrome
Acromegaly

Hypothalamic Lesions -- Tumors
Infection
Idiopathic
Infiltrative disorders (sarcoid, histiocytosis)

Chest wall manipulation (manual, surgery, trauma, infection)

Endocrine -- Cushings disease, Acromegaly

Chronic Renal Disease -- decreased clearance of prolactin.

Tumor with ectopic secretion of prolactin.

Diagnostic Plan: Eliminate drugs associated with elevated prolactin.
Serum prolactin level (levels > 100 associated with pituitary adenomas).
TSH level -- rule out thyroid disorders
MRI/CT scan of head when prolactin levels elevated.

Treatment: Based on etiology --
1) Discontinue drug use if this is the cause.
2) Treat underlying hypothroidism.
3) Microadenomas: bromocriptine --
Follow prolactin levels q 6 months
Repeat MRI/CT scan in 6 months, then q 2 - 3 years
4) Macroadenoma: Surgical removal if mass effect is present or bromocriptine --
Follow prolactin levels q 6 months.
Repeat MRI/CT scan q 6 months.

Scrotal Disorders

Scrotal Swelling and Masses

History:
> Pain -- abrupt onset suggests torsion.
> Trauma
> Change in testicular size.
> Sexual activity: epididymitis is rare without sexual activity.
> Prior history of pain: torsion may be preceded by episodes of mild pain.

Examination:
> Inspection: 1 testes higher than other suggests torsion, infected testes often lower.
> Palpation: If pain alleviated by scrotal elevation, consider epididymitis or orchitis. No change in pain, suspect torsion.
> Painless masses: Asses location; tumor associated with testes.
>> Varicocele : "bag of worms" on left spermatic cord.
>> Spermatocoele or hydrocele: mass near epididymitis
>> Transilluminate: clear -- hydrocele
>>> spermatocele
>> absence -- suggests tumor

Laboratory:
> UA: Pyruia > 20 WBC/hpf (edididymitis)
> Gram stain: Gram negative diplococci suggests epdidymitis. Negative gram stain suggests chlamydial epididymitis, orchitis or torsion.
> Doppler and scans: Doppler flow study crucial in suspected torsion. If not available, surgical exploration is indicated. Flow will be decreased to torsed testicle.

Differential Diagnosis:
> Painless scrotal mass or swelling:
>> Hydrocele
>> Spermatocele
>> Varicocele -- prevalence 5 - 15% in 10 - 20 year age group.
>> Hernia
>> Testicular tumor -- 2.3/100,000 maleu, rish increased with history of cryptorchism.
>> Idiopathic scrotal edema
> Painful scrotal mass or swelling:
>> Torsion of spermatic cord
>> Epididymitis
>> Orchitis
>> Trauma -- hematoma
>> Hernia
>> Torsion of testicular appendage

Management:
> Torsion: Immediate surgery within 6 hours of symptom onset.
> Epididymitis: Scrotal support
>> Bedrest
>> Ceftriaxone and Doxycycline (cover for gonorrhea and chlamydia)
>> Refer to urologist if symptoms do not resolve.
> Testicular tumors (most common solid tumor in mases 15 - 35 years old):

Biopsy for confirmative diagnosis and cell type.
Definitive therapy based on biopsy.
Hydrocele: No therapy unless --
1) tense hydrocele reduces circulation to the testes.
2) bulky mass is uncomfortable or uncosmetic.
Definitive therapy is resection of the parietal tunica vaginalis.
Varicocele: No therapy unless --
1) condition is painful.
2) massive distention exists.
3) involved testis is significantly smaller than the other.
Spermatocele: No therapy indicated.

SEXUALLY TRANSMITTED DISEASES IN ADOLESCENTS

Disease /Organism	Clinical Presentation	Diagnosis	Treatment	Complication/Sequelae
Nongonococcal Urethritis -- chlamydia trachomatis -- ureaplasma urealyticum	Males: Dysuria Frequency Mucoid to purulent urethral discharge. Some asymptomatic.	WBC'S on gram stain of discharge. + chlamydia FA/culture - gonorrhea culture	Doxycycline, Tetracycline, or Erythromycin for 7 days Refer/rx partner Use condoms	Urethral strictures Prostatitis Epididymitis
Mucopurulent Cervicitis -- chlamydia trachomatic -- N. gonorrhea -- Herpes simplex virus	Females: Asymptomatic or yellow mucopurulent endocervical exudate	Exudate on endocervical swab > 20 PMNs/HPF on gram stain of endocervical discharge. + chlamydia culture/FA + GC culture	Ceftriaxone I.M. or Cefixime P.O. PLUS Doxycycline or Erythromycin Refer/rx partner Use condoms	Salpingitis PID Conjunctivitis, pneumonia in newborn.
Gonorrhea	Males: Dysuria, purulent urethral discharge. Females: Vaginal discharge, abnormal menses, lower abdominal pain, asymptomatic. Look for pharyngeal and rectal infection.	Microscopic indentification of gm negative Diplococci on urethral exudate or endocervical material. Positive culture.	Ceftriaxone I.M. or Cefinime P.O. and Doxycycline or Erythromycin	PID Epididymitis Sterility

PID
(Pelvic inflammatory disease)
	Females: Pain, tenderness in lower abdomen, cervix, uterus, adnexa.
	
	Fever, chills, increased sed rate, WBC.
	
	Hx: multiple sexual partners, past history of PID, IUD.
	
	R/O ectopic pregnancy, appendicitis
		Definitive visualization of inflamed fallopian tubes and positive culture of tubal exudate at laparoscopy.
		
		Presumptive -- clinical presentation +/- positive cultures.
			Outpatient:
			Cefoxitin/Probenecid or Ceftriaxone PLUS Doxycycline or Erythromycin for 14 days
			
			Inpatient
			Doxycycline BID
			   PLUS
			Cefoxitin I.V. q 6
			      OR
			Clndamycin PLUS Gentamycin.
				1) Ectopic pregnancy
				
				2) Abscess
				
				3) Involuntary infertility
				
				4) Recurrent PID
				
				5) Recurrent Pelvic Pain

Condylomala Acuminala (congenital warts) Human papilloma virus	Single or multiple soft, fleshy growths on perineum, perianally on cervix, intravaginally.	Visual culposcopy PAP smear	Cryotherapy Podophyllin (not in pregnancy) TCA Electrocautery Examine sexual partner	Obstruction of vagina Infection of newborn Cervical cancer
Herpes Genitalis (Herpes Simplex Virus, Types I and II)	Single or Multiple vesicles of genitalia. Rupture leads to painful ulcers	Presumptive history, typical lesions, multinucleated giant cells on PAP smear Definition: HSV tissue culture showing cytopathic effects	No Known Cure Palliative: Acyclovis with 1st episode Annual PAP smears	Fetal Wastage infection of newborn. Urethral stricture
Syphilis Treponema Pallidum	Primary -- classical chancre is painless, indurated. suspect syphillis in all genittal lesions Secondary -- skin rash (palms and soles) Condyloma lata, Lymphadenopathy Latent -- 0 clinical signs	Presumptive -- Primary: typical lesion and newly positive serologic test, or titer of serologic test for syphilis 4 fold greater that last titen. Secondary: presentation and strongly reactive serological test. Definitive: + dark field examination of material from lesion or lymphnode.	Primary, Secondary, early Syphylis < 1 year: Benzathne Penq. or if allergic to Pen - use Doxycycline or Erythromycin Rx partner	Congenital Syphilis Cardiovascular Syphilis Neurologic involvements
Chancroid Hemophillis ducreys	Single, superficial painful ulcer, inguinal bubo (25 - 60%)	presumptive -- clinical presentation (R/O syphilis) Definitive -- culture + for H. ducreys	Erythromycin or Ceftriaxone	Secondary infection of ulcer Buleoes may rupture causing fistula.
Molluscum Centagiosum (DNA virus from Poxvirus group)	1 - 5mm smooth rounded shiny, firm, papule, with unbilicated centers	presentation -- microscopic exam of maternal from lesion reveals molluscum inclusive bodies	Curettage Cryotherapy	secondary infection
Pediculosis pulas phthirus pubis (pubic louse)	itching, erythematous papules, nits or adult lice on pubic hairs	Exam -- lice or nits on pubic hair	Lindane, clean linen in hor water. Treat partner.	Excoriation lymphadermitis pyoderma

Reproductive Issues

Half of all adolescents sexually active by 17 years of age. < 1/3 use any effective form of birth control.

Contraception:
    Oral Contraceptive Pill -- Most common form used by adolescents.
        Failure rate 2 - 4%.

        Mechanism of Action -- Suppresses ovulation, decreases likelihood of
            implantation, makes cervical mucus hostile to sperm.

        Contraindications to use in adolscents --
            Absolute -- Hypertension
                History of thromboembolic disease, cerebrovascular
                  accident.
                Undiagnosed abnormal genital bleeding.
            Relative -- Borderline hypertension
                Migraine headaches
                Diabetes
                Sickle Cell Disease
                Cigarette smoking

        Common side effects --
                Breakthrough bleeding.
                Nausea
                Weight gain
                Headaches
                Mood swings

        Advantages -- Decreased menstrual flow
            Decreased dysmenorrhea
            Improvement of acne

        Evaluation prior to starting Pill --
                Screen for risk factors
                Complete physical examination
                Pelvic examination
                Weight and blood pressure check
                Laboratory PAP smear, gonorrhea culture, chlamydia FA or
                  culture, RPR and pregnancy test if indicated.

    Barrier Methods -- used by < 20% of adolescents.
        Failure rate 10 - 20%.

        Mechanism of action -- Prevent sperm from entering uterus

        No contraindications to use.

        Types -- Diaphragm
            Cervical Cap
            Condom

    IUD -- not usually recommended in sexually active teenagers.

    Injectible Pregesterone -- most commonly used contraception outside the United
        States.

Mechanism of action -- suppresses ovulation

Indications for use -- significant contraindication to estrogen use exists.
Patient unwilling to use barriers contraceptives or the pill.
When all other forms of contraception have failed and pregnancy is not desired.
Adolscent is mentally unable to understand the meaning of pregnancy and is unable to use other forms of contraception.

Acne
major skin problem in adolescents

Pathophysiology:
Androgens produced during puberty cause increased sebum production form the sebaceous gland. Bacteria in the follicles attract a white leukocyte response. WBC activity then releases hydrolytic enzymes which cause a local inflammatory reaction. Resolution may leave scarring.

Definition of lesions:
Comedo - hyperkeratosis of follicular epithelium.
Whiteheads - closed comedones resulting in elevated papules in the skin.
Blackheads - later stage of enlarged comedones that contain malanin; when they eventually open, it leads to inflammatory changes.
Cystic acne - not cysts; they are composed of nodules resulting in erythematous papules (pimples) or pus-filled papules (pustules).

Treatment: - goal is to decrease sebum production and decrease bacterial activity.
Comedolytic and antikeratolytic agents:
topical retinoic acid
benzoyl peroxide
Antibacterial agents:
topical and systemic antibiotics (tetracycline)
Sebaceus gland inhibitior:
systemic isotretinoin
oral contraceptives
Surgical removal of comedones and scars
Exfoliating agents:
ultraviolet light
cryotherapy

Mental Health Issues

Depression

60% of teenagers surveyed said they experienced depression once a month to daily
More common in women than men.

Etiology: change in peer and/or dating relationships.
family influences, problems with parents.
poor school experiences: bad grades, conflict with teachers, peer conflict.
poor self image.

Clinical features: Recurrent somatic complaints.
Mood swings.
Decline in school performance.
Apathy.

Therapy: Counseling for family and teenager.
May consider antidepressant, but be cautious.

Suicide:

3rd most common cause of death in adolescents.
Suicide attempts outnumber sucessful suicides 50-200/1.
Women make more attempts.
Males more often succeed.
60% of teenagers who commit suicide have made a previous attempt.

Preventive steps:
1) All adolescents should be asked about suicidal thought.
2) If suicidal thoughts are present assess risk
- review history of suicide/suicide attempts
- assess level of family support and recognition of problem
- teenager recovering from depression is more likely to commit suicide
- danger signs:
getting affairs in order
giving things away
withdrawal from family/friends
history of suicide or alcohol abuse in family
- precipitating events:
break-up with significant other
conflict with peers
pregnancy
conflict with parents (most common)

Therapy: Team approach - physician, social worker, psychiatrist.
Ambulatory treatment
- no significant past history
- method used less lethal
- suicide attempt occurred when help was available
- family is supportive and recognizes problem
- mental health care worker is available
- patient and family willing to follow-up
Hospitalization necessary:
- safe environment needed

- family not supportive
- past history of suicide attempt
- history of depression
- method used was lethal or medical care needed
- attempt occurred without warning
- ambulatory services not available

Substance Abuse

Stages:

Stage I - Experimentation
Starts with peers, under peer pressure.
Few behavioral changes.
User experiences euphoria and guilt.

Stage II - Abuse to relieve stress
More than occasional use.
Occurs in nonsocial settings.
Supply of substance maintained.
Peer group develops around substance abuse.

Stage III - Regular abuse
User involved in drug-oriented culture.
Most peers use drugs. Problem behavior chronic.
May have trouble with the law.
User depressed when not using drugs.
User needs to raise money to support habit.

Stage IV - Dependence
Drug used to prevent drpression not to produce euphoria.
Adolescent may drop out of school.
Physical changes such as weight loss, fatigue, blackouts and
chronic cough may occur.

Therapy: Stages I and II may be treated on an outpatient basis.
Stages III and IV require hospitalization and/or placement in
residential rehabilitation facility.

Thomas A. Lera
A. Eugene Osburn

Developmental Considerations

The concept of a syndrome was originally used to describe a constellation of findings that recurred from individual to individual without recognized underlying cause. Describing something as a syndrome is useful because it affords prognostic information about a patient with the constellation of findings. The approach to genetics was originally to classify recognizable patterns of congenital malformations and subsequently identify chromosomal abnormalities that were associated with them. This led to a focus on individual genes carried on chromosomes and identification of diseases arising from defects in individual genes. Knowledge of modes of inheritance based on the characteristics of the gene allowed prognostication about appearance of the disease in offspring of affected parents, and the acquired knowledge of mechanisms of disease offered new opportunities for therapeutic intervention. Modern molecular genetic methodologies use a reverse approach. The defective gene is identified first through techniques of gene mapping and then its effect on the biologic processes is elucidated. The techniques which allow gene mapping also allow synthesis of replacement fragments for defective genes and potentially their incorporation into the genetic matrix of the affected individual via recombinant DNA technology (genetic engineering). Future information on the results of these activities may reflect changes in the direction of medical knowledge and intervention as much as any other current research activity.

Genetics addresses the mechanisms by which genes serve as templates for cell structure and function, and how the information in such genes are transmitted to newly generated cells (or, in the case of gamate cells, to new individuals). Each normal human diploid cell contains all its genetic information in 23 pairs of chromosomes. Of these, 22 pairs are autosomal chromosomes, and one pair is the sex chromosome. Each autosomal pair of chromosomes is composed of a complementary chromosome (haploid) from each parent. Analogous genes in the matching chromosomes are called alleles. If a single copy of the gene (a single allele) pair can exert an effect alone, it is called a dominant gene. If an effect is detectable only when two identical alleles are present, the gene is termed recessive. Individuals who have two identical alleles for a gene are homozygous and those with two different alleles are heterozygous. Individuals with a heterozygous allele for a recessive gene are carriers for the trait regulated by the recessive gene.

X-linked inheritance is modified by the nature of the X chromosome. Males have only one X chromosome and will express any gene on the X chromosome, including sex-linked recessive genes such as hemophilia A. Genes on the Y chromosome of the male sex chromosome pair do not appear to be active other than for determining maleness. Females have two X chromosomes. Which of the two is active in which cells is determined by a phenomenon called mosaicism.

Genetic characteristics of genes are expressed in offspring through **Mendelian inheritance patterns**:

Autosomal dominant inheritance
Autosomal recessive inheritance
Sex-linked inheritance

Pedigree analysis

A pedigree analysis for an inherited condition can be used to infer the mode of inheritance of the condition.

Autosomal dominant conditions have a 50% chance of being passed to any one offspring.

In autosomal recessive conditions, only 25% of the offspring born to unaffected parents would be expected to inherit the one recessive gene from each parent necessary for the condition to be expressed.

Many autosomal recessive disorders effect enzymes or proteins that transport metabolites. Heterozygous individuals have enough of the enzyme to survive, but the homozygous individual may not and may present with clinical features of an inborn error of metabolism.

Many conditions which tend to run in families cannot be explained by strict Mendelian inheritance patterns alone. These are designated multifactorial disorders.

Dysmorphology

Dysmorphology is a subset of genetics which studies structural development abnormalities.

Birth defects can be the result of sporadic factors, single gene disorders, chromosomal disorders, teratogens, or multifactorial disorders.
Malformations are the result of abnormalities in tissue formation;
Deformations are the result of insults to normally formed tissues in utero;
Disruption is the complete breakdown of previously normal tissue in utero.

Inborn Errors of Metabolism

Clinical deterioration of a previously normal neonate should suggest the possibility of an inborn error of metabolism. Their presentation in this age period is similar to that of neonatal sepsis. The infant can be normal at birth because of support from the mother via placental exchange of critical metabolic pathway components.

Diagnostic Modalities

DNA analysis:
    Can be used to identify single gene disorders such as hemophilia A, muscular dystrophy, sickle cell anemia, thalassemia, congenital adrenal hyperplasia and phenylketonuria.

Enzyme assay:
    Can be used to identify defective enzymes or the metabolites they regulate.

Chromosome analysis:
    Can be used to confirm suspected cases of Trisomy 13, 18, 21, Turner syndrome, Kleinfleter syndrome, Fragile X, and chromosome deletions.

Alpha-fetoprotein levels:
    Elevated in: Twins, neural tube defects, intestinal obstruction, congenital hepatitis, congenital nephrosis, impending fetal demise.
    Decreased in: Trisomy 21

Ultrasonography:
    Useful for detection of gross structural defects.

Chorionic villus biopsy:
    Can be performed between 8 to 11 weeks gestation to obtain samples for numerous assays. Used only in situations where fetal risk outweigh possible benefit from information gained.

Lipoprotein electrophoresis
Four major classes of lipoproteins can be separated by electrophoresis techniques:

Chyolmicrons
    Mostly triglycerides. Produced in the intestine from dietary fat.
Very low-density lipoproteins (VLDL)
    Predominately triglycerides. Synthesized in the liver. Catabolized to LDL.
Low-density lipoproteins (LDL)
    Predominately cholesterol. LDL specific receptors are required for them to be transported into cells for utilization.
High-density lipoproteins (HDL)
    Predominately cholesterol. Derived from chylomicrons and VLDL in the liver and intestine. High levels are protective from coronary heart disease.

HbA$_{1C}$

Hemaglobin A$_{1C}$ is a measurement of glycosylated hemaglobin and is an indicator of the prevailing glucose concentration in the blood. The higher the concentration of serum glucose and the longer the RBC hemoglobin has been exposed to it the higher the percent of Hemaglobin A$_{1C}$ which is expressed as a percent of normal hemoglobin. Normal HbA$_{1C}$ in non diabetics is less than 7%; levels above 12% in diabetics indicates poor control of the diabetes.

Pathophysiologic Manifestations

Representative Autosomal Dominant Diseases

Achondroplasia
Gilbert disease
Hereditary hemorrhagic telangiectasia
  (Osler-Weber-Rendu disease)
Hereditary spperocytosis
Huntington disease
Hyperlipidemia
Marfan syndrome
Myotonic dystrophy
Neurofibromatosis
Protein C deficiency
Tuberous sclerosis
von Willebrand disease

Representative Autosomal Recessive Diseases

Alpha-1-antitrypsin deficiency
Congenital adrenal hyperplasia
Cystic fibrosis
Galactosemia
Gaucher disease
Glycogen storage diseases
Mucopolysaccaridoses (MSD)
  (all MSD's except Hunter syndrome, which is X-linked)
Phenylketonuria
Sickle cell anemia
Tay-Sachs disease
Wilson disease

Representative X-linked Diseases

Bruton agammaglobulinemia
Color blindness
Duchenne muscular dystrophy
Fragile X syndrome
Hemophilia A + B
Lesch-Nyhan syndrome

Viable Autosomal trisomy chromosomal disorders

Trisomy 13
Trisomy 18
Trisomy 21

Sex chromosome disorders

Syndrome	Defect
Turner syndrome	Female: single normal X chromosome
Klienfelter syndrome	Male: extra X chromosome
Fragile X syndrome	Male: fragile site on long arm of X chromosome

Approach to Inborn Errors of Metabolism in the Neonatal Period

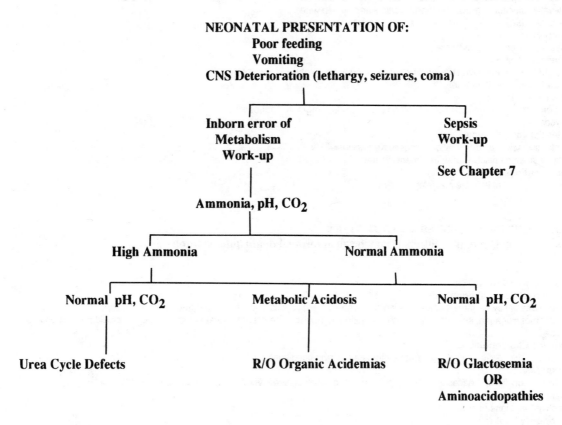

NEONATAL PRESENTATION OF:
Poor feeding
Vomiting
CNS Deterioration (lethargy, seizures, coma)

Inborn error of Metabolism Work-up

Sepsis Work-up

See Chapter 7

Ammonia, pH, CO_2

High Ammonia

Normal Ammonia

Normal pH, CO_2

Metabolic Acidosis

Normal pH, CO_2

Urea Cycle Defects

R/O Organic Acidemias

R/O Glactosemia
OR
Aminoacidopathies

Endocrine Disorders

INSULIN DEPENDENT DIABETES MELLITUS, TYPE I
Most common endocrine-metabolic disease in childhood
Etiology
unknown
Pathophysiologic abnormality
Decreased glucose utilization and increased glucose production
Elevated glucagon, growth hormone, cortisol and epinephrine
Lipolysis, fatty acid mobilization and keto acid production
Symptoms
polyuria, polyphagia, polydipsia
Physical findings
weight loss invariable in children if untreated, increased height may result form
growth hormone stimulation.
Laboratory findings
hyperglycemia (a verifiable random blood glucose > 200 mg/dl is diagnostic)
glycosuria
Potential complications
Metabolic acidosis, dehydration, Diabetic Ketoacidosis
Hypoglycemic episodes after treatment initiated.
Therapeutic plan
Insulin replacement is the mainstay of therapy

INSULIN DEPENDENT DIABETES MELLITUS, TYPE II
This condition is rare in children. It may be an autosomal dominant condition.

DIABETIC KETOACIDOSIS
Pathophysiologic abnormality
Insulin deficiency or unresponsiveness which causes hyperglycemia and intracellular depletion of glucose. This stimulates production of glucagon, epinephrine, growth hormone and cortisol. The result is accelerated lipolysis, keto acid production and acidosis.
Predisposing conditions
missed insulin doses, infections or other stress producing conditions
Symptoms
polyuria, polydipsia, headache, lethargy, fatigue, dehydration, nausea, vomiting, abdominal pain
Physical findings
Tachypnea, signs of dehydration
Laboratory findings
elevated glucose, elevated WBC, dilutional hyponatremia, elevated BUN, decreased bicarbonate
Potential complications
dehydration, cerebral edema
Therapeutic plan
insulin, volume expansion, correction of ketosis and acidosis, replinish potassium

HYPERTHYROIDISM
Alternate terminology
Graves' disease, thryotoxicosis
Etiology
Autoimmune disorder causing hyperfunctioning of the thyroid gland via stimulation of thyrotropin receptors most common. Other causes are rare in children.
Predisposing conditions
Girls 4:1 more common than boys, Onset before 5 years rare; usually in adolescence. Family history of Graves' disease or Hashimoto's thyroiditis
Symptoms
decline in school performance,weight loss, emotional lability, frequent loose stools, sleep disturbance, weakness
Physical findings
hyperactive, proptosis, enlarged thyroid gland, wide pulse pressure, resting tachycardia, proximal muscle weakness, tremor of fingers
Laboratory findings
increased T_4, increased T_3 resin uptake, decreased TSH
Chronologic sequence of manifestations

insidious onset and progression
Potential complications
thyroid storm
Theraputic plan
propylthiouracil (PTU) or methimazole; subtotal thyroidectomy; radioactive iodine
Prognosis

CONGENITAL HYPOTHYROIDISM
Alternate terminology
Cretinism
Etiology
thyroid agenesis, ectopic thyroid, maternal thyroid abalation treatment
Symptoms
lethargy, prolonged neonatal jaundice, refractory constipation
Physical findings
hypotonia, large open fontanelle, coarse facies, thick enlarged tongue, hoarse cry, umbilical hernia, developmental delay, heart murmurs, pedal edema
Laboratory findings
decreased T_4, decreased T_3 resin uptake, elevated TSH, decreased bone age by X-ray
Potential complications
severe permanent neurologic impairment
Therapeutic plan
neonatal screening, thyroid hormone replacement with L-thyroxine
Prognosis
good, if detected and effectively treated before 3 months of age

JUVENILE HYPOTHYROIDISM
Etiology
chronic lymphocytic thyroiditis (Hashimoto's thyroiditis), goitrogens, overtreatment of hyperthyriodism
Predisposing conditions
more common in girls
Symptoms
decreased linear growth, delayed puberty, lethargy, constipation, cold intolerance
Physical findings
coarse facies, sluggish movement, delayed DTR's dry, thin hair, pale, waxy skin
Laboratory findings
decreased T_4, decreased T_3 resin uptake, elevated TSH, decreased bone age by X-ray
Potential complications
myxedema, other autoimmune disorders if etiology due to autoimmune mechanism
Therapeutic plan
L-thyroxine replacement
Prognosis
good if treated

CONGENITAL ADRENAL HYPERPLASIA
Alternate terminology
Adrenogenital syndrome
Etiology
90% are due to 21-hydroxylase deficiency
Pathophysiologic abnormality
in 21-hydroxylase deficiency, there is an accumulation of its' precursor 17-hydroxyprogesterone; cortisol and aldosterone deficiencies
Predisposing conditions
Symptoms
vomiting, dehydration, shock developing in first 2-4 weeks of life
Physical findings
Females have ambigous genitalia; males are normal
Laboratory findings
hyponatremia, hyperkalemia, metabolic acidosis, hypoglycemia; elevated serum 17-hydroxyprogestetone
Differential diagnosis
presentation may suggest **pyloric stenosis**, but that has **hypokalemia and a metabolic alkalosis**
Theraputic plan
Cortisol replacement and mineralcorticoid to supress plasma renin level

A. Eugene Osburn

Developmental Considerations

A host defense system helps ensure the homeostasis of the human organism by providing protection against infection, malignancy and autoimmune diseases. Some of the defense system is static, such as the skin barrier and mobile cilia. Others are able to adapt to challenges presented to the organism as "foreign substances". The major components of the adaptive system of defense are the T lymphocytes, B lymphocytes, phagocytes and the complement system.

Undifferentiated stem cells in the fetal bone marrow and liver give rise to three cell lines, which differentiate according to the microenvironment in which they mature. Stem cells which migrate to the thymus and develop under the influence of local humoral factors become T-Cells. Those which migrage to the bone marrow become B-Cells and enter the circulation to populate lymphoid follicles.

B-Cells

B-Cells differentiate into plasma cells which secrete immunoglobulins. The classes of and functions of immuglobulins are:

IgM: adult levels are produced by 1 year of age
10% of immunoglobulins pool
Forms rapidly after antigenic stimulation
Aids in opsonization and agglutination

IgG: adult levels are produced by 5-7 years of age
70-75% of immunoglobulin pool
Protect against bacteria, viruses and fungi
Major antibody of rechallenge immume responses
Persists after antigenic stimulation
Crosses placenta in latter half of 3rd trimester

IgA: adult levela are produced by 10-14 years of age
15-20% of immunoglobulin pool
Secretory antibody in saliva, lacrimal fluid and colostrum,
   nasal secretions, bronchial secretions and intestinal
   secretions

IgD: less than 1% of immunoglobulin pool
Serves as receptor site on circulating B cells

IgE: small amount of immunoglobulin pool
Found on surface of mast cells and basophils
Allergic individuals often have high serum levels

T-Cells

T cells function as regulators and amplifiers of the immunologic response of other immunocompetent cells. They release soluable mediators (lymphokines) in response to appropirate antigenic challenge which in then recruit macrophages, granulocytes and other immunocompetent cells. Some of the T cells are cytotoxic cells and can lyse target cells selectively. Helper T cells have a surface antigen marker termed CD4 and suppressor (cytotoxic) T cells have a CD8 surface antigen.

Phagocytes

Phagocytes are able in ingest and then destroy engulfed mircoorganisms, and are able to migrate toward a chemical stimulus initiated by an inflammatory response. Mast cells and basophils are mediators of the immediate hypersensitiviy response. The have receptors with a high affinity to IgE but can be activated by non IgE mechanisms. Upon activation, they secrete mediators of an inflammatory response within seconds, the most prominent being histamine.

Complement system

Components of the complement system are involved in the inflammatory response in both effector and regulatory functions. There are two pathways of complement activation: the classic and the alternative. Either leads to activation of a common final pathway, which results in formation of a membrane attack complex. The classic pathway is initiated by IgG or IgM antigen-antibody complexes; the alternative pathway does not require antibody for its activation. C3 is consumed as the first component of either pathway. Regularory proteins modulate the activity of complement. Alternative pathway activation occurs only as a result of loss of inhibition mediated by these regulatory proteins. Most bacteria cells lack activators of these inhibitors. However, bacteria rich in sialic acid - such as group B Streptococcus, Neisseria and E. Coli - are able to resist alternative pathway activation and therefore are more pathogenic in individuals who lack sufficient antibody activatiors of the classic pathway (e.g. neonates).

Diagnostic Modalities

Laboratory tests for Immune Competence

Screening tests

General
- CBC with Differential
- X-rays, bone scans to identify infections
- Cultures as indicated
- Erythrocyte sedimentation rate

Tests of antibody mediated (humoral: B-cell) immunity
- Quantitative immunoglobulin levels of IgG, IgM, IgA, IgE
- Isohemagglutinin titer (anti-A, anti-B) to measure IgM function
- Patient's antibody response to immunization to diphtheria, tetanus toxoid and measles-mumps-rubella vaccine

Tests of cell-mediated (T-cell) immunity
- Absolute lymphocyte count
- Delayed hypersensitivity skin tests to Candidia, tetanus toxoid, tuberculin and mumps

Tests of phagocytosis mediated immunity
- Absolute neutrophil count
- Nitroblue tetrazolium (NBT) dye test to measure neutrophil metabolic function
- IgE level

Tests of complement mediated immunity
- Total hemolytic complememt (CH50) to measure complement activity
- C3, C4 levels to measure important pathway components

Advanced immunologic tests

Antibody
- HIV antibody
- B cell quantitation
- IgG subclasses
- Secretory antibody levels
- Pre-existing antibody levels: measles, polio, diphtheria, tetanus
- Specific antibody response: pneumococcal, H. influenzae

Cell-mediated
- T-cell quantitation and subpopulations
- Mitogen stimulation response
- Mixed lymphocyte culture assays
- Thymic hormone assays

Phagocyte
    Rebuck skin window for chemotaxis
    Chemotaxis, adhesion, aggregration assays
    Enzyme assays: myeloperoxidase
    Metabolic assays: chemiluminescence
    Phagocytic and bactericidal assays

Complement
    Classic pathway individual component assays
    Alternative pathway individual component assays
    C1 esterase inhibitor
    Chemotatic factors
    Opsonic assays

Pathophysiologic Manifestations

Clinical characteristics of B Cell Defects

Recurrent pyrogenic infections with extracellular encapsulated organisms
    (e.g. Pneumonococcus, H. Influenzae, streptococcus)
Otitis, sinusitis, recurrent pneumonia, bronchiectasis, conjuncitivitis
Diarrhea, especially due to Giardia lamblia infection
Decreased serum immunoglobulins

Growth is usually normal
Increased rate of viral and fungal infections are rare
    (except for enterovirus encephalitis and poliomyelitis)

Prognosis: survival to adulthood, or years after onset

Clinical characteristics of T Cell Defects

Recurrent infections with opportunistic or less virulent organisms
    (e.g. viruses, fungi, protozoa, mycobacteria)
Maladsorption, diarrhea, growth retardation, failure to thrive
Anergy
Graft-versus-host reaction if given non irradiated blood
Live virus vaccinations or BCG vaccinations can be fatal
High incidence of Malignance

Prognosis: survival beyond infancy or childhood is rare

Clinical characteristics of Phagocytic Defects

Recurrent skin infections with bacteria and fungi
> (e.g. Staphlococcus, Pseudomonas, E. Coli and Aspergillus)

Abscesses of lymph nodes, subcutaneous tissue, liver and lung
> (pulmonary infections are common and contribute to chronic lung disease)

Bone and joint infections are common

Clinical characteristics of Complement Defects

Recurrent bacterial infections with extracessular pyogenic organisms
> (e.g. pneumococcus, H. influenzae)

Unusual susecptibility to recurrent neiserria infections
> (e.g. Gonoccus and Meningococcus)

Increased incidence of autoimmune disease
> (e.g. SLE, rheumatoid arthritis, sarcoidosis)

Recurrent or severe skin and respiratory tract infections

Causes of secondary immunodeficiencies

Premature and newborn infants

Infections
> Bacterial, viral (AIDS, Epstein-Barr virus), fungal , tuberculosis

Neoplastic Disease
> Leukemia, Hodgkin disease, nonlymphoid cancer

Surgery and trauma
> Burns, splenectomy, stress

Autoimmune Disease
> SLE, Rheumatoid arthritis, Graft-versus-host disease

Protein-losing States
> Protein losing-enteropathy, nephrotic syndrome

Immunosuppresive Treatment
> Chemotherapy, radiation therapy, corticosteroids

Hereditary and Metabolic Diseases
> Malnurtition, uremia, diabetes mellitus, sickle cell anemia,
> chromosomal abnormalities

Disease Profiles

Selected Primary Immunodeficiency Disorders

Disorder	Clinical Manifestations	Inheritance
B cell		
X-linked agammaglobinemia (Bruton's)	Recurrent pyogenic infections of the CNS, sinuses, middle ear, lungs and skin	X-linked
Dysgammaglobulinemia IgA deficiency IgM deficiency IgG subclass deficiencies unknown	Recurrent infections of sinses, lungs; gastrointestinal disease	Variable AR
Common variable immunodeficiency unknown	Infections of sinuses, middle ear, lungs; giardiasis; malabsorption; autoimmune disease	AR, AD,
Transcobalamin II deficiency	Recurrent infections; megaloblastic anemia; intestinal villous atrophy; defective granulocytic bactericidal activity	AD
T cell		
Wiskott-Aldrich syndorme	Eczema; thrombocyopenia; recurrent infections; malignancy	X-linked
DiGeorge syndrome unknown	Hypoparathyroidism; facial abnormalities; cardic abnormalities; predisposition to mental deficiency and gastrointestinal tract malformations	
Ataxia-telangiectasia	Oculocutaneous telangiectasia; progressive cerebellar ataxia; bronchiectasis; malignancy	AR
Severe combined immunodeficiency	Recurrent infections; chronic diarrhea; failure to thrive	X-linked AR

Hypersensitivity reactions

Mechanisms which provide host defense can also cause tissue damage if the reaction is exaggerated. Four major types of reaction are recognized:

Type I hypersensitivy reaction
anaphylactic, atopic or reaginic reaction
mediated by IgE triggered release of histamine and other substances
Examples: hay fever, extrensic asthma, anaphylatic shock

Type II hypersensitivy reaction
antibody mediated cytotoxic reaction
IgG or IgM binds to cell carried antigens resulting in lysis
Example: autoimmune hemolytic anemia

Type III hypersensitivy reaction
Immune-complex mediated reaction with tissue deposition
complement activation is involved
Examples: autoimmune diseases, serum sickness, Arthus reactions

Type IV hypersensitivy reaction
Sensitized T-cells bind to cellular antigens and result in lysis
Examples: Graft rejection, contact dermatitis

In situations where the host defense mechanisms do not recognize the individuals own cell antigens as not foreign, autoimmune diseases arise. The most common mediators of autoimmune diseases are misdirected type II and type III hypersensitivity reactions. Some of the arthritic and connective disorders which may be due to such mechanisms are:

Systemic lupus erythematosus
Rheumatoid arthritis
Rheumatic fever
Lyme disease
Serum sickness
Mucocutaneous lymph node syndrome (Kawasaki disease)
Henoch-Schonlein purpura
Atopic dermatitis/Eczema

A. Eugene Osburn

Developmental Considerations

Cancer is the second most common cause of death in children between 1 and 15 years of age.

The most common types of cancers in children, in decreasing order of frequency, are:

Leukemia
Central nervous system tumors
Lymphoma
Neuroblastoma
Soft tissue sarcoma
Wilm's tumor
Bone tumors
Retinoblastoma
Others

Most cancers in children are still of unknown etiology. The postulated candidates for causing a malignant transformation in normal cell lines is similar to those postulated for birth defects involving structural or metabolic derangements:

Genetic propensities
Environmental agents
Altered immunogenicity
Some viral infections

Pathophysiologic Manifestations

Signs and symptoms suggestive of cancer
> Prolonged fever
> Night sweats
> Weight loss
> Abdominal masses
> Thoracic masses
> Painless lymphadenopathy
> Bone pain
> Petechiae
> Signs of increased intracranial pressure
> Ataxia
> Exophthalmos
> Proptosis
> Leukokoria

Therapeutic Options

Surgery
Radiation therapy
Chemotherapy
Bone Marrow Transplant

Disease Profiles

LEUKEMIA
Etiology
  Classification:
        Acute (97% of childhood leukemias)
           Acute lymphocytic leukemia (80% of acute childhood leukemia)
           Acute nonlymphocytic leukemia (20% of acute childhood leukemia)
        Chronic (3% of childhood leukemias)
           all chronic leukemias in childhood are nonlymphocytid
Pathophysiologic abnormality
  Bone marrow replacement by leukemia cells resulting in anemia, hemorrhagic diathesis, susceptablity to infection and bone pain; reticuloendothelial system infilration resulting in hepatosplenomagalyand lymphadenopathy
Predisposing conditions
  immunodeficiency states, solid tumors, congenital bone marrow failure
Symptoms
  pallor, irritability, fatigue, fever, symptoms of infection, bone pain
Physical findings
  lymphadenopathy, hepatosplenomagaly, petechiae, echymoses, signs of infection
Laboratory findings
  anemia, thrombocytopenia, neutropenia, blast cells in periphreal smear (can be missed by automated cell counters); bone marrow examination: diagnostic cell morphology
Potential complications
  hyperuricemia, hyperkalemia, complications of RBC, platelet and functional WBC's; tissue infiltration
Diagnostic plan
  bone marrow aspiration
Therapeutic plan
  Antileukemic therapy dependent on type of leukemia
Prognosis
        Favorable prognostic indicators:
           age 2-7 years
           White
           Female
           Initial WBC < 10,000
           Normal IgG, IgM, IgA
           Non-T, non-B cell ALL

CENTRAL NERVOUS SYSTEM TUMORS
Second most common form of childhood cancer (20% of total childhood cancers)
Etiology
  Classification:
        Tumors of Astrocytic orgin
           High-grade astrocytomas (arise above tentorium)
           Low-grade astrocytomas (arise below the tentorium in the cerebellum)
           Brain stem gliomas
        Tumors of Neuroepithelial orgin
           Medulloblastoma
           Primitive neuroectodermal tumors
Pathophysiologic abnormality
  mass lesion causing focal neurologic deficits and increased intracranial pressure
Symptoms
  symptoms of increased intracranial pressure; symptoms due to focal neurologic involvement
Physical findings
  Signs of increased intracranial pressure; focal neurologic deficits; ataxia and nystagmus if lesion below tentorium
Diagnostic plan
  MRI of head; CT with contrast material
Theraputic plan
  Surgical resection, chemotherapy and radiation therapy are all used, but all have potential serious side effects

NEUROBLASTOMA

Second most common solid tumor in childhood (brain tumor is most common solid tumor)

Pathophysiologic abnormality

malignancy of neural crest cells; signs and symptoms depend on whether tumor is in the head and neck, chest or abdomen

Predisposing conditions

infants and preschool children: half are under 2 years of age

Laboratory findings

elevated vanillymandelic acid (VMA), elevated homovanillic acid (HMA)

Diagnostic plan

Establish staging:

Stage I: localized

Stage II: does not cross midline

Stage III: tumor crosses midline

Stage IV: metastatic dissemination

Stage IVS: in young infants with metastasis to skin, liver, bone marrow, but not cortical bone

Theraputic plan

surgical resection for stages I, II and IVS; chemotherapy

Patrice A. Aston
A. Eugene Osburn

Developmental Considerations

Infants under 2 to 3 months of age are not able to isolate and localize infections very effectively. Also, they may not at that age show signs of infection other than temperature changes - either fever or hypothermia. Therefore, infants under 2 months age with a rectal temperature over 38.5 C, or who are hypothermic should have a "Sepsis Workup" and be started on IV antibiotics until the culture results indicate it is safe to stop them.

Even if their temperature is less than 38.5, infants under 2 months of age who are found to have an infection which is presumably due to a bacterial cause (e.g. pneumonia, otitis media, UTI), should be assumed to be incapable of localizing the infection, and started on IV antibiotics after a "Sepsis Workup" is done. For example, the finding of concurrent meningitis requires a longer course of antibiotics than does otitis alone.

Maternal placentally transfered immunity lasts a few months. Because it does, it influences when immunizations should be begun in the infant.

A child's temperature is normally lower in the early morning than late in the afternoon after they have been active. The maximal daily temperature of children usually occurs between 5:00 and 7:00 PM.

Excessive clothing can interfer with the child's ability to dispate normal body heat and raise it's tempetature.

A normal homeostatic mechanism establishes the temperature threshold in children at around 41.1 C (106 F).

Leukocytes have greater phagocytic activity at 38 to 40 C than at lower temperatures.

Fever per se does not cause convulsions. Febrile seizures occur in 5% of children, and the seizure occurs during the rise in temperature. Thus, if a child has a high fever for hours or days, he/she will not suddenly have a convulsion because of the fever alone. If the underlying cause of the fever is something which irritates the CNS, such as meningitis, then a seizure may occur, but it is the meningitis which causes the convulsion, not the fever.

Children in day care get more URI,s for their age than those exposed to fewer contacts. The extent to which those children later in their school years have fewer URI's because they have already acquired an immunity to the agents causing URI's is not known.

Because of it's association with Reye's syndrome in children and adolescents, aspirin should not be used to treat fever in these groups.

There is no such thing as a "Viral Syndrome". Fever in a child with an unrecognized cause does not necessarily mean the child has a viral infection.

Diagnostic Modalities

Gram stain
Useful for classifying bacteria and thus narrowing the list of diagnostic possibilities. Organisms with recognizable structures such as some fungi and parasites can be identified without staining.

Cultures
Bacterial and Fungal
Selective media is used to classify the bacteria or fungus as to type and subtype. This information can then be used to guide selection of a theraputic agent.

Viral
Viral cultures are usually done in tissue cultures. This method can take significantly longer than that available for bacteria and fungi.

Immunologic techniques
Immunofloresence
Florescent antibodies (FA) are specific antisera are used to identify some bacteria by the typical fluorescence that results when they are added to sera containing the suspected organism.

Agglutination tests
A substance, usually latex, is coated with antibodies that will agglutinate when added to sera containing their antigen.

Countercurrent immunoelectrophoresis (CCIE)
Is able to detect antigens in body fluids, including CSF and urine. It can identify antigens of H. influenzae type b, S. Pneumonia, and some types of N. Meningitidis. The latex agglutination is more sensitive and can also detect antigens of group B streptococcus.

ELISA
enzyme-linked immuno-sorbent assay is used to detect viral antibodies. It is now available for detecting most viruses. For HIV it is both sensitive and specific, but not absolutely certain, so confirmatory tests (e.g. Western blot) must be done.

Beta-lactamase production can be determined for staphylococci, *Haemophilus influenzae* and Neisseria gonorrhoeae. Its presence means a resistence to penicillin and ampicillin by the bacteria.

The Sepsis Work Up

A sepsis workup is done when a significant infection is feared and and either an obvious source or the extent of the infection is not evident. It is a constellation of procedures selected to optimize identification of the cause and extent of the infection, since these can influence selection of appropriate treatment. The components of the septic work up are:

Blood Cultures
> A minimum of one blood culture is obtained

Lumbar Puncture
> CSF is sent for: Protein, Glucose, Culture and Sensitivity, CCIE, Cell Count, and other studies based on clinical suspicion

Chest X-Ray
> Obtained to rule out pneumonia, as well as other chest pathology

Chem 7 (Na, K, Cl, CO_3, Glucose, BUN, Cr)
> The glucose is needed for compairson with the CSF glucose, BUN and Cr to assess hydration status and guide dosing of potentially nephrotoxic drugs, Electrolytes provide guidance in fluid therapy and assess the potential of Inaproprate ADH found in some cases of meningitis (especially H. Influenza)

Urine
> For Culture and Sensitivity as well as routine studies. It should be obtained by suprapubic tap in infants under 3 months of age

WBC: the white blood count can be supportive, but is not diagnostic of a bacterial infection. Typically the WBC is elevated in bacterial infections and normal or decreased in viral infections. However, early viral infections may have elevated WBC's and overwhelming bacterial may cause a decreased number of WBC's. Also other conditions such as leukemia can obscure the interpretation of the WBC.

(CAUTION: an automated blood cell counter can not differerentate between blast cells and lymphocytes and will report them as lymphocytes or monocytes)

Focus of the Physical Examination in febrile children

REGION	FOCUS	SIGNIFICANT ABNORMALITIES
General Appearance		
	Playfulness	Disinterest in activities or play
	Interactiveness	Withdrawn demeanor
	Alertness	Aware of those in the room
	Consolability	Unresponsive to comforting
	Irritability with movement	Movement of inflamed tissue, including the meninges, causes pain
	Color	Pallor or Cyanosis
	Hydration	Sunken eyes or fontanel dry mucous membranes
HEENT		
	Fontanelle	Bulging or Depressed
	Nuchal rigidity	Brudsenski and Kernig signs
	Rhinorrhea	Purulent discharge may be due to sinusitis
	Tympanic Membranes	Erythemia, lack of mobility
	Drooling	Found in severe pharyngitis, gingivostomatitis, retropharyngeal abscess, and epiglottitis
Heart		
	Murmurs	New onset in Rheumatic Fever, endocarditis
	Friction Rubs	Suspect precarditis
	Distant Heart Sounds	Suspect pericardial effusion
Lungs		
	Persistent cough	Suspect pneumonia, especially in the infant
	Expiratory grunting	Suspect pneumonia
	Subcostal or intercostal Retractions	Respiratory distress
	Flaring of nasal alae	Respiratory distress
Abdomen	Localized tenderness	Appendicitis, hepatitis, pyelonephritis
Extremeties	Joint swelling, pain	Septic joint, arthritis
	Bone pain	Osteomyelitis, Leukemia, Sickle Cell Crisis
Integument	Petechial Rashes cellulitis	Meningococcemia, Rocky Mountain Spotted Fever, Leukemia

Pathophysiologic Manifestations

Fever. There are literally hundreds of diseases which have fever as one of its components. Since there are so many, the finding of fever **alone** does not narrow the list of diagnostic possibilities much.

A decrease in temperature after adminstration of antipyretics does not distinguish between bacterial and viral infections.

General Causes of Fever
Infections
Vaccines
Drugs
Collagen-vascular diseases
Inflammatory diseases
Tissue injury
Granulamotous diseases
Endocrine disorders
Malignancy
High environmental temperatures
CNS lesions affecting the hypothalmus/brain stem
Anhydrotic ectodermal dysplasia
Dehydration
Strenous exercise
Factitious fever

Summary of selected bacterial infections by age groups

SITE	Most common pathogens	Intital treatment
Sepsis/Meningitis		
< 2 months	group B streptococci	ampicillin and cefotaxime
	E. coli	or
	Listeria monocytogenes	ampicillin and gentamicin
	N. meningitidis	
	S. pneumoniae	
2 months - 8 years	*H. influenzae*	cefotaxime (or ceftriaxone
	N. meningitidis	or cefuroxime) or
	S. pneumoniae	ampicillin and chloramphenicol
> 8 years	*N. meningitidis*	*penicillin G*
	S. pneumoniae	
Acute Otitis Media		
< 2 months	*S. pneumoniae*	ampicillin and gentamicin
	H. influenzae	or
	group A streptococci	or
	S. aureus	cefotaxime
	gram negative enteric	
2 months - 8 years	*S. pneumoniae*	Amoxicillin or
	H. influenzae	erythromycin/sulfisoxazole or
	B. catarrhalis	augmentin or
	group A streptococci	cefaclor or
	S. aureus	cefixime
> 8 years	*S. pneumoniae*	Penicillin V or
	group A streptococci	erythromycin
Pneumonia		
< 2 months	group B streptococci	erythromycin (if afebrile)
	S. aureus	*ampicillin and gentamicin*
	Chlamydia trachomatis	or
	S pneumoniae	ampicillin and cefotaxime
2 months - 8 years	*S. pneumoniae*	*amoxicillin or*
	H. infulenzae	erythromicin/sufisoxazole or
	S. aureus	cefaclor or cefixime or
	mycoplasma	augmentin
> 8 years	*S pneumoniae*	erythromycin
	mycoplasma	

Urinary tract infection

< 2 months	Assume neonatal sepsis until proved otherwise	
> 2 months	*E. coli* *Proteus* species *Klebsiella* species *Staphlococcus epidermidis* *Enterococci*	ampicillin (or amoxicillin) or trimethoprim/sulfamethaxazole or cephalexin (or cefaclor) or sulfisoxazole or nitrofurantoin

Osteomylitis

all age groups	S. aureus S. pneumoniae	base on culture and sensitivity
< 5 years sickle cell patients puncture wound of foot	H. influenzae salmonella Pseudomonias aerginosa	

Septic Joint

< 2 months	S. aureus group B streptococcus gram negative enteric	nafcillin and gentamicin
2 months - 8 years	H. influenzae S. aureus Streptococcal species	nafcillin and ceftriaxone
> 8 years	S. aureus Neisseria gonorrhoeae	nafcillin and ceftriaxone

Febrile patients at increased risk for infectious causes

Patient group	At risk for
Neonate < 1 month old	Group B streptococcus, *E. Coli, Listeria monocytogenes*, herpes simplex
Infant < 3 month old	Group B streptococcus, *E. Coli, Listeria monocytogenes*, respiratory syncytial virus, enterovirus, *H. influenzae*, N. mengitidis
Temperature > 41 C	Meningitis, bacteremia, pneumonia, Heat stroke, hemorrhagic shock-encephalopathy syndrome
Petechial rash with fever	Meningococcus, *Haemophilus influenzae type b*, pneumococcus, Rocky Mountain Spotted Fever
Sickle cell anemia	Pneumococcal sepsis, meningitis, Salmonella
Asplenia	Encapsulated bacteria, esp. pneumococcus, Salmonella
Agammaglobuinemia	Bacteremia, sinopulmonary infection
AIDS	Pneumococcus, *H. influenzae type b*, Salmonella
Immunosuppressive drugs	*Pseudomonas aeruginosa, S. aureus, Candida, S. epidermidis*
Left to right shunt heart lesions	endocarditis
Central venous lines	*S. aureus, S. epidermidis, Cornebacteria, Candida*

Childhood Exanthems

Disease	Incubation period	Typical distribution	Clinical features
Maculopapular lesions			
Measles (Rubeola)	10 - 14 days	Begins at hairline and descends downward; Generalized by 3rd day; Confluent on face, neck, upper trunk	3 day prodrome with 3 C's: Cough, Conjunctivitis, Coryza; Koplik's spots 2 days before rash; desqumates after 7-10 days
Rubella (German measles, 3 day measles)	14 - 21 days	Begins on face, progresses rapidly downward; Generalized by second day; Fades in order of appearance	Postauricular, suboccipital lymphadenopathy; Arthirtis common in women
Roseola (exanthema subitum)	10 - 14 days	Appears after defervescence of fever; initially on chest, then face, extremeties; fades rapidly	3-4 day prodrome of high fever in otherwise well appearing 1 to 4 year old child
Erythema infectiousum (Fifth disease; caused by parvovirus B19)	7 - 14 days	Red flushed cheeks with circumoral pallor (slapped cheek); followed by reticular, lacy rash on extremities; may recur on exposure to trauma, sunlight, heat	Patients with diseases that shorten RBC life span may have an aplastic crisis
Enterovirus (especially Echovirus type 9)	few days	Rubella like lesions; nonpuritic; may be petechial; lasts 3-5 days	Fever, malaise, sore throat, rhinorrhea, vomiting, diarrhea, herpangina; illness may mimic meningococcemia
Scarlet fever (Group A streptococci)	2 - 4 days	Sandpaper texture; appears 1st on flexor surfaces, then generalized; most intense on neck, shoulders, axila, inguinal, popliteal skin folds, circumoral pallor, lasts 7 days then desqumates	Pharyngitis, tonsilitis, strawberry tongue, palatal petechiae
Vesicular/pustular lesions			
Varicella (Chickenpox)	14 - 21 days	Discrete puritic macules which progress to vesicles, umbilicated pustules and then crusted lesions; all stages are present at the same time; can involve mucous membranes	Avoid aspirin. Contagious until all lesions are crusted over.
Herpes zoster (shingles)		Erythemia followed by red papules, then vesicles in 12-24 hours, then pustules in 72 hours, then crusts in 10-12 days; unilateral periphreal dermatome distribution; does not cross midline	History of varicella Preeruptive pain common
Hand, foot and mouth syndrome (Coxsackievirus A16)	4 - 6 days	Palmar and plantar pustules have typical eliptical football shaped appearance	Fever, myalgia, malaise, herpangina, rhinorrhea, vomiting, diarrhea
Desmiinated gonococcemia		Erythematous or hemorrhagic papules that evolve into pustules or vesicles with an erythematous halo	Affects primarily young women; Fever and migratory polyarthralgias are commen
Impetigo (group A streptococcus; bullous lesions are caused by stophylococci)		Honey colored crusted lesions with predilection for face and exposed areas; bullous lesions are round bullae which rupture quickly	Poststreptococcal glomerulonephritis is potential complication; Bullous impetigo may be mistaken for cigatette burns
Insect bites		Local reactions may resemble infectious exanthems or may be secondarily infected	

Disease Profiles

Systemic Infections

OCCULT BACTEREMIA

Presence of bacteria in the bloodstream with out clinical mainfestations other than fever.

Etiology

S. pneumoniae, H. influenzae type b, N. meningitidis, Group A streptococcus, S. aureus

Predisposing conditions

age 6 months to 2 years

Symptoms

fever (usually > 102), irritablilty

Laboratory findings

WBC > 15,000, low colony count positive blood culture

Diagnostic plan

blood culture, CBC

Therapeutic plan

if not S pneumonia, treat as sepsis

Prognosis

spontaneous resolution in 24 to 48 hours with S.pnerumoniae, sepsis with others

SEPSIS

Life threatening invasion of the bloodstream which may seed local areas.

Etiology

H. influenzae and N. meningitidis, and S. pneumonia ore most common

Predisposing conditions

compromised host defense, immaturity

Symptoms

high fever, local pain (if invasive)

Physical findings

petechial rash

Laboratory findings

WBC > 15,000 with shift to left, Positive blood culture

Potential complications

meningitis, osteomyelytis, septic joint

Diagnostic plan

septic work up

Therapeutic plan

age dependent: see table above

Central Nervous System Infections

MENINGITIS

Inflammation of the meninges

Etiology

bacterial, aseptic, fungal, atypical bacterial

Pathophysiologic abnormality

inflammation of the meninges

Symptoms

severe headache, altered sensorium, seizures, vomiting

Physical findings

meningeal signs (nuchal rigidity, Kernig's or Brudzinski's signs) bulging fontanelle, seizures

BACTERIAL MENINGITIS

Etiology

age specific: see table above

Pathophysiologic abnormality

usually hematogenously seeded

Laboratory findings

Elevated CSF WBC's, Elevated CSF protein, decreased CSF glucose, positive CSF culture and gram stain, positive latex agglutination test, positive CCIE

Potential complications

shock, DIC, subdural effusion, cerebral edema, seizures, SIADH, neurologic sequelae

Diagnostic plan

sepic work up

Therapeutic plan

age specific: see table above

ASEPTIC MENINGITIS

Non bacterial inflammation of the meninges

Etiology

Viruses
  Enteroviruses (85% of cases)
   coxsackie virus
   echoviruses
  Arboviruses
   St. Louis encephalitis virus
   California encephalitis virus
  HIV
  varicella
  Epstein-Barr virus
  lymphocytic choriomeningitis
  measles
  rubella
  rabies
  influenza
  parainfluenza
  CMV
  mumps
Mycoplasma
chlamydia
Various fungi, protozoa and other paracytes
postinfectious reactions to various viruses
  Less common causes include: leptospirosis, syphilis, Lyme disease, Cat-scatch fever, nocardiosis, Rocky Mountain spotted fever, vasculitis, intracranial hemorrhage, reactions to NSAIDS and heavy metal poisoning

Symptoms

headache, irritibility,fever, nausea, vomiting, retrobulbar pain

Physical findings

nuchal rigidity, exanthems, signs of underlying disease

Laboratory findings

elevated CSF WBC's (often predominately polymorphoneucular cells early, lymphocytes and mononuclear cells later), Normal or slightly elevated CSF protein, normal CSF glucose in viral causes, negative CSF gram stain

Therapeutic plan

supportive, if viral cause

Prognosis

usually self limiting if viral cause

ENCEPHALITIS

An acute inflammation of brain parenchyma

Etiology

herpes simplex, St. Louis encephalitis virus, California encephalitis virus, eastern equine encephalitis virus, western equine encephalitis virus,coxsackie virus, echoviruses; postinfectious encephalitis following measles, mumps, varicella, rubella; Mycoplasma pneumonia, Toxoplasma gondii

Symptoms
similar to aseptic meningitis, but more severe CNS manifestations: confusion, delirium, hallucinations, memory loss, combativeness, seizures and coma

Physical findings
focal neurologic signs: ataxia, signs of increased intracranial pressure

Laboratory findings
increased CSF RBC's with herpes simplex; increased CSF WBC's (usually 10 - 500), increased CSF protein, normal CSF glucose

Diagnostic plan
Brain biopsy may be indicated if herpes simplex is suspected

Therapeutic plan
Acyclovir for herpex simplex and complicated herpes zoster; other eitologies generally supportive care for increased ICP

Prognosis
St. Louis , California, western equine encephalitis: good
eastern equine, herpes simplex encephalitis: 60% death, high incidence of serious neurologic sequelae

Facial Infections

PERIORBITAL CELLULITIS

Etiology
H. influenzae, streptococcus, pneumococcus

Symptoms
no pain with movement of eyes

Physical findings
inflammation of eyelids and periorbital tissues; no proptosis

Potential complications
orbital cellulitis

Differential diagnosis
trauma, periorbital edema, local allergic reactions

Therapeutic plan
oral antibiotics to cover likely etiologic agents; careful monitoring to detect progression to orbital cellulitis

Prognosis
good if non progressive

ORBITAL CELLULITIS

Etiology
H. influenzae, streptococcus, pneumococcus

Symptoms
pain with movement of eyes, fever

Physical findings
inflammation of eyelids and periorbital tissues; proptosis; chemosis

Laboratory findings
leukocytosis

Potential complications
cavernous sinus thrombosis; meningitis; epidural, subdural or brain abscess

Diagnostic plan
septic work up

Therapeutic plan
IV antibiotics

BUCCAL CELLULITIS

Except for the location, the implications of this entity parallel those of periobrital cellulitis

Oral Infections

APTHOUS STOMATITIS

Alternate terminology
canker sores

Etiology
uncertain, may be infectious

Symptoms
painful local buccal leisons

Physical findings
painful shallow circular ulcers on buccal mucosa

Differential diagnosis
exanthem of other vrial illnesses

Therapeutic plan
symptomatic; topical antibiotic barrier

Prognosis
self limiting in 1 to 2 weeks, recurrent

CANDIDAL GINGIVOSTOMATITIS

Alternate terminology
thrush

Etiology
Candida species,usually candida albicans

Predisposing conditions
common in infants, if occurs after after infancy, consider immune deficiency

Symptoms
decreased feeding in infants

Physical findings
grayish white lesions on buccal mucosa and dorsum of tongue

Laboratory findings
pseudohyphae on gram stain, candidia on culture

Therapeutic plan
nystatin oral suspension

HERPETIC GINGIVOSTOMATITIS

Alternate terminology
cold sores

Etiology
herpes simplex; usually type I, may be type II

Pathogenesis
primary infection involves the mouth and gums, recurrent infections the lips

Pathophysiologic abnormality
after primary infection the virus lies dormant in nerve tissue until reactivated

Predisposing conditions
recurrence is precipitated by stress, either physical or emotional

Symptoms
fever to 105, painful lesions

Physical findings
erythematous, edematous, ulcerative lesions in mouth

Chronologic sequence of manifestations
Incubation period 3-9 days; improves after 3-10 days; resolves in 2 weeks

Potential complications
dehydration

Therapeutic plan
cold foods and liquids, mixture of Maalox and Benadryl, analgesics, IV fluids sometimes needed

HERPANGINA

Alternate terminology
Hand, foot, mouth when characteristic lesions are also on those locations

Etiology

Coxsackie virus types A & B; echoviruses
Symptoms
headache, myalgia, fever, sore throat, dysphagia, vomiting
Physical findings
temperature to 106, ulcerative lesions on posterior pharynx, tonsilar pillars and soft palate
Chronologic sequence of manifestations
fever lasts 3-5 days, lesions may last a week
Potential complications
dehydration
Therapeutic plan
symptomatic, cool foods and liquids, analgesics

NECROTIZING ULCERATIVE GINGIVITIS
Alternate terminology
Vincents stomatitis, trench mouth
Etiology
fusiform bacilli and spirochetes invading areas of interdental papillae eroded by plaque
Predisposing conditions
severe dental plaque
Physical findings
fever, maloderous breath, gingival pain
Therapeutic plan
penicillin G

Upper Respiratory Infections

SINUTITIS
Etiology
S pneumonia, unencapsulated strains of H. influenzae, B. catarrhalis
Pathophysiologic abnormality
frontal sinuses are not developed until school age maxiallary sinusitis rare before 18 months
Predisposing conditions
allergic rhinitis, URI, swimming, trauma,
Symptoms
fever, headache, chronic rhinorrhea, maloderous nasal discharge, persistent cough
Physical findings
purulent rhinorrhea, periorbital swelling, localized tenderness, maloderous breath
Laboratory findings
sinsus X-ray: air fluid levels, opacity of sinus
Potential complications
orbital cellulitis, meningitis, brain abscess, cavernous sinus thrombosis
Therapeutic plan
amoxicillin

ACUTE OTITIS MEDIA
Alternate terminology
suppurative otitis media if membrane is perforated
Etiology
S. pneumonia, unencapsulated H. influenzae, B. catarrhalis, Group A streptococcus, S. aureus
Predisposing conditions
eustachian tube dysfunction leading to adsorption of air from middle ear leaving a vacuum
Symptoms
URI symptoms, ear pain, fever, hearing impairment, vomiting, diarrhea
Physical findings
erythematous, bulging, non mobile TM
Potential complications
hearing deficit with impaired language acquistion

Therapeutic plan
amoxicillin

STREPTOCOCCAL PHARYNGITIS
Etiology
group A beta hemolytic streptococcus
Symptoms
fever, sore thoat, headache, abdominal pain
Physical findings
fever, exudative tonsillar hypertrophy, petechiae on soft palate, tender anterior cervical nodes
Laboratory findings
positive rapid strep screen, positive culture
Potential complications
otitis media, acute sinusitis, peritonsillar abscess, cervical lymphadenitis, acute rheumatic fever, acute glomerulonephritis
Differential diagnosis
viral pharyngitis, Corynebacterium diphtheriae, M. pneumonia, Infectious mononecleuosis, N. gonorrhoeae opportunitic infections in leukemia
Diagnostic plan
rapid strep screen, throat culture
Therapeutic plan
penicillin p.o. for 10 days

VIRAL PHARYNGITIS
Etiology
Epstein-Barr virus, adenovirus, herpes simplex virus, enterovirus, influenza virus, parainfluenza virus, measles
Symptoms
indistinguishable from strep. pharyngitis
Physical findings
indistinguishable from strep. pharyngitis
Therapeutic plan
symptomatic

INFECTIOUS MONONEUCLEOSIS
Etiology
Epstein-Barr virus
Symptoms
malaise, headache, fever, sore throat, fatigue, abdominal pain
Physical findings
pharyngitis, tender anterior and posterior cervical nodes, splenomegaly, maculopapular rash
Laboratory findings
positive monospot test, antibodies to EBV
Potential complications
splenic rupture, hepatitis, airway obstruction, aseptic meningitis, Guillain-Barre syndrome
Therapeutic plan
avoid contact sports until spleen normal

ACUTE EPIGLOTITIS
Etiology
H. influenzae type b
Pathophysiologic abnormality
infectious edema of the epiglottis
Predisposing conditions
age 2-7 years, lack of Hib vaccine
Symptoms
rapid onset: fever, sore throat
Physical findings
respiratory distress, stridor, drooling, sitting forward with mouth open, cherry red epiglottis (should only be viewed in Operating Room)
Laboratory findings
lateral soft tissue neck X-ray: characteristic Thumb

sign

Chronologic sequence of manifestations
symptoms and findings evolve in hours from none to life threatening

Potential complications
complete airway obstruction

Differential diagnosis
visualization under controlled conditions should not be delayed by diagnostic tests

Diagnostic plan
transport to an Operating Room where ansthesiology and ENT personel are available; avoid aggitation

Therapeutic plan
Endotracheal intubation; ventilatory support; IV antibiotics to cover Beta lactimase producing organisms

Prognosis
good if airway controlled and antibiotics effective

ACUTE LARYNGOTRACHEOBRONCHITIS

Alternate terminology
viral croup

Etiology
respiratory viruses; parainfluenza most common

Pathophysiologic abnormality
laryngeal edema

Symptoms
hoarseness, barking cough, fever, URI symptoms

Physical findings
inspiratory stridor, respiratory distress

Laboratory findings
Lateral neck soft tissue X-ray: subglottic narrowing (penciling)

Chronologic sequence of manifestations
symptoms progress over days; often worse at night

Therapeutic plan
humidified air; racemic epinephrine if hospitalized; corticosteriods

Lower Respiratory Infections

BRONCHIOLITIS

Etiology
respiratory syncytial virus (50%); parainfluenza virus; adenovirus

Pathophysiologic abnormality
infectious edema of bronchiolar mucosa; bronchospasm is not a component

Predisposing conditions
rare after 2 years age

Symptoms
cough, wheezing, dyspnea, feeding difficulty

Physical findings
wheezing, flaring of nasal alae, crackles; may have cyanosis

Laboratory findings
rapid viral antigen assays

Chronologic sequence of manifestations
mild URI symptoms followed by progression of respiratory distress

Potential complications
apnea, respiratory failure

Differential diagnosis
Asthma (rare under 9 months), foreign body aspiration, pertussis, CHF, pneumonia

Diagnostic plan
pulse oxymeter, chest X-ray

Therapeutic plan
Ribavirin if due to RSV and illness is severe

Prognosis
may be prone to asthma later in life

PNEUMONIA

Etiology
Bacterial, viral, fungal, rickettsiae agents

Pathophysiologic abnormality
infection of lung parenchyma

BACTERIAL PNEUMOMIA

Etiology
S. pneumonia, H. influenzae type b, Group A streptococcus

Symptoms
abrupt fever, shaking chills, cough, chest pain

Physical findings
crackles, decreased breath sounds, flaring of nasal alae, grunting respirations

Laboratory findings
consolidation on chest X-ray; leukocytosis; blood cultures may be positive

Therapeutic plan
age specific; see table above

VIRAL PNEUMONIA

Etiology
RSV most common; other respiratory viruses

Theraputic plan
Ribavirin for severe RSV or influenza pneumonia
Acyclovir for severe herpesvirus pneumonia

MYCOPLASMA PNEUMONIA

Etiology
M. pneumoniae

Predisposing conditions
peak age: 5-15 years

Symptoms
sore throat, non productive cough, fever, headache, malaise

Physical findings
may have few signs

Laboratory findings
cold agglutinins positive; chest X-ray: interstitial infiltrate

Therapeutic plan
erythromycin

P. CARINII PNEUMONIA

Etiology
P. carinii

Predisposing conditions
immune compromised patient

Symptoms
exertional dyspnea is characteristic in older patients; severe respiratory distress with cyanosis in infants

Laboratory findings
tracheal washings positive

Therapeutic plan
trimethoprim-sulfamethoxazole

Cardiac Infections

ENDOCARDITIS

Etiology
Alpha-hemolytic streptococcus, S aureus, S. epidermidis

Pathology

Pathogenesis

Pathophysiologic abnormality
Predisposing conditions
central venous lines, IV drug abuse, valvular heart
lesions, cardiac shunts with high turbulence
Symptoms
fatigue, fever, malaise
Physical findings
Roths spots, Janeway lesions and Osler's nodes are
rare; changing murmurs, splinter hemorrhages
Laboratory findings
positive blood cultures; vegitations seen on echo
Potential complications
emboli, mycotic aneurysms, CHF
Therapeutic plan
long term IV antibiotics (at least 4 weeks)

MYOCARDITIS
Etiology
enteroviruses (coxsackie,B, echovirus)
Symptoms
fever, symptoms of CHF
Physical findings
dysrhymthias, signs of CHF, abnormal EKG
Laboratory findings
EKG: ST segment depression, T-wave inversion;
Chest X-ray: cardiomegaly, pulmonary vascular
congestion, edema
Potential complications
Coxsackie myocarditis is extremely sensitive to
digitalis; regular digitalizing doses can be highly toxic
Therapeutic plan
supportive treatment
Prognosis

PERICARDITIS
Etiology
Bacteria, viruses, fungi and tuberculosis
Pathophysiologic abnormality
inflammation with fluid accumulation in the pericardial
sac
Symptoms
left shoulder pain, back pain, relieved by sitting
forward, fever, cough, dyspnea
Physical findings
pericardial friction rub, distant heart sounds
Laboratory findings
echo: pericardial fluid; chest X-ray: enlarged heart with
normal pulmonary vascularity; EKG: ST segment
elevation
Potential complications
cardiac tamponade
Therapeutic plan
pericardical drainage, antibiotics if bacterial etiology

Gastrointestinal System Infections

HEPATITIS A
Alternate terminology
infectious hepatitis
Etiology
HV virus
Symptoms
may be mistaken for a cold in children; fever, RUQ
pain, anorexia, nausea, vomiting, diarrhea
Physical findings
Jaundice, hepatomegaly, RUQ tenderness
Laboratory findings
elevated liver transaminases, elevated direct and

indirect bilirubin, positive hepatitis A-IgM indicates
acute disease
Chronologic sequence of manifestations
incubation period: 2-6 weeks; prodromal phase may
not be noticed in children; GI symptoms, dark
urine, jaundice subsides after 1-2 weeks
Potential complications
fulminant hepatitis
Differential diagnosis
infectious mononeucleosis, leptospirosis, CMV,
Wilson's disease, other viral hepatitis
Therapeutic plan
supportive meaures; enteric isolation
Prognosis
generally good in children
Prevention
exposed household contacts should get IgG within 2
weeks of contact

HEPATITIS B
Alternate terminology
serum hepatitis
Symptoms
fever, arthralgia, RUQ pain, anorexia, nausea,
vomiting, diarrhea
Physical findings
Jaundice, hepatomegaly, RUQ tenderness
Laboratory findings
elevated liver transaminases, elevated direct and
indirect bilirubin, positive hepatitis B surface antigen
(HB_sAg) indicates acute disease; antibodies against
the hepatitis B surface antigen (HB_sAb) indicates
immunity; presence of HB_eAg indicated infectivity
Chronologic sequence of manifestations
incubation period: 2-6 months; GI symptoms, dark
urine, jaundice subsides after 1-2 weeks
Potential complications
fulminant hepatitis, carrier state, chronic active
hepatitis (predisposes to hepatocellular carcinoma)
Differential diagnosis
infectious mononeucleosis, leptospirosis, CMV,
Wilson's disease, other viral hepatitis
Therapeutic plan
supportive meaures; enteric isolation
Prognosis
generally good in children
Prevention
HBV vaccine

Urinary Tract Infections

CYSTITIS
Etiology
E. coli, other intestinal organisms
Predisposing conditions
female, anatomic abnormalities
Symptoms
dysuria, urgency, frequency
Laboratory findings
positive urine culture
Potential complications
pyelonephritis
Therapeutic plan
oral antibiotics

PYELONEPHRITIS
Symptoms
gastrointestinal symptoms common, fever, chills, flank
pain
Physical findings

CVA tenderness
Potential complications
hypertension, renal insufficency if severe renal damage
Therapeutic plan
IV antibiotics if toxic

Joint Infections

SEPTIC JOINT
Alternate terminology
septic arthritis
Etiology
S aureus: often preceded by trauma
H. influenzae: most common in children < 5 years; often associated with infection elsewhere, e.g. meningitis, otitis media
Streptococci: group A, B, anaerobic, Streptococcus viridans
S. pneumonia
N. gonorrhoeae: primarily hands, wrist, knee, ankle
gram negative enteric: neonates, immunosuppressed
Pseudomonas organisms: immunosuppressed, neonates, puncture wounds
Pathophysiologic abnormality
bacterial invasion of joint space
Symptoms
fever, irritability, joint pain, may appear toxic
Physical findings
joint effusion, swelling, limitation of motion
Laboratory findings
ESR elevated, blood cultures positive (50% of time), WBC may be elevated
Joint aspirate: WBC > 50,000, Glucose < 50% of blood glucose; poor mucin clot
x-ray: bone demineralization (late finding) joint distension
Bone scan: Technetium: positive within 24 hours may be able to differientiate osteomylelitis
Gallium: positive within 24-48 hours; becomes normal with effective treatment
Potential complications
destruction of cartilage, growth plate
Differential diagnosis
see chapter on musculosleletal disorders
Therapeutic plan
see table above for antibiotic choices
Surgical drainage often required
Prognosis
better the sooner effective treatment is begun

Bone Infections

OSTEOMYELITIS
Etiology
similar to septic joint plus mycobacteria and in immunocompromised patients, fungal
Pathology
Pathogenesis
Pathophysiologic abnormality
predeliction for metaphysis of long bones
Predisposing conditions
trauma, systemic bacterial infection, immunocompromised host, sickle cell disease, drug abuse
Symptoms

fever, local pain; infants may have little systemic toxicity
Physical findings
local warmth, swelling, tenderness; limp; restricted movement
Laboratory findings
WBC may be elevated; ESR elevated; blood culture positive > 50% of patients
X-ray: soft tissue swelling in 3-4 days; bone changes in 7-10 days (periosteal elevation, lytic changes, sclerosis)
Bone scan: technetium most helpful
Potential complications
chronic osteomyelitis; septic joint; growth plate damage
Differential diagnosis
septic arthritis, cellulitis, fracture, Ewing's tumor
Therapeutic plan
see table above

Disseminated infections

ROCKY MOUNTAIN SPOTTED FEVER
Etiology
Rickettsia rickettsii
Pathophysiologic abnormality
diffuse vasculitis
Predisposing conditions
tick bite
Symptoms
fever, chills, headache, irritability, confusion, delirirm, myalgia, photophobia
Physical findings
conjunctivitis, profuse nonpitting edema, rash: rose colored macules beginning on wrists, hands, ankles and feet (involves palms and soles), then becoming petechial and purpuric over entire body
Laboratory findings
hyponatremia, thrombocytopenia, positive immunoflorescence antibody
Chronologic sequence of manifestations
abrupt onset after 2- 8 day incubation period
Potential complications
neurologic deficits, coma, renal failure, DIC, gangrene of distal extremeties, shock
Differential diagnosis
see meningococcemia
Therapeutic plan
tetracycline or chloramphenicol

MENINGOCOCCEMIA
Etiology
Neisseria meningitidis
Symptoms
fever, headache, malaise, arthralgia, vomiting
Physical findings
pink maculopapular rash; generalized petechiae, including palms and soles; (if purpura and ecchymosis expect high mortality)
Laboratory findings
scraping of purpuric lesion may have positive gram stain and culture
Chronologic sequence of manifestations
onset insidious to fulminant; may progress to death in 12 hours or less
Potential complications
meningitis; pericarditis, DIC, Waterhouse-Friderichen

syndrome, cardiovascular collapse, death
Differential diagnosis
 rocky mountain spotted fever, H. influenzae (rarely),
 leukemia, idiopathic hrombocytopenic purpura,
 infectious mononucleosis, measles, Henoch-Schonlein
 purpura, viral infections
Therapeutic plan
 penicillin IV; respiratory isolation
Treatment of contacts
 rifampin

ACQUIRED IMMUNE DEFICIENCY SYNDROME
 Alternate terminology
  AIDS
 Etiology
  Human T lymphotropic virus type III (HLTV-III); also
  referred to as human immunodeficiency virus (HIV)
 Pathology
 Pathogenesis
 Pathophysiologic abnormality
  OKT 4 positive lymphocytes ore infected, causing cell
  dysfunction, immune deficiency and cell death. AIDS
  results when opportunistic infections supervene.
  common opportunistic infections include: P carinii
  pneumonia, Candida esophagitis, disseminated
  cytomegalovirus, cryptosporidiosis, chronic herpes
  simplex virus nfections, cryptococcosis, toxoplasmosis,
  mycobacterium avium intracellulare
 Predisposing conditions
  exposure to HIV positive body fluids
 Symptoms
  reflective of underlying opportunistic infection:
   Infants: failure to thrive
   Older children: AIDS-related complex (ARC) with
   hepatomegaly, lymphadenopathy, chronic diarrhea,
   recurrent infections, neurologic deficits are common.
 Laboratory findings
  screening HIV positive by ELISA; confirmed by western
  blott assay, HIV culture, positive HIV antigen
 Chronologic sequence of manifestations
  HIV infection, ARC, AIDS
 Potential complications
  cardiomyopathy, nephropathy, Neurlolgic deficits,
  growth failure, eventual death from oportunistic
  infections
 Diagnostic plan
  CBC with differential;
  T cell evaluation: delayed skin hypersensitivity,
   T cell subset assay, mitogen and antibody
   stimulated lymphocyte blastogenesis
  B cell evaluatlion: quantitative immunoglobulins,
   B cell enumeration
 Therapeutic plan
 supportive treatment; Azidothymidine (AZT)

A. Eugene Osburn

Developmental Considerations

Infants are obligate nasal breathers. Complete occulsion of the nares can result in life threatening apnea. Nasal obstruction can also interfer significantly with feeding in older infants since it is difficult to maintain an effective suck without a patent nares.

In evaluating the symptoms of respiratory diseases in infants, remember to investigate the possibly of symptoms due to over the counter cold remedies. Sleep disturbances, irritibility, etc. may be a side effect of the medication, not a manifestation of the condition it was given for.

Airway resistance to airflow is inversely proportional to the fourth power of the radius of the airway. Therefore, a given degree of tissue swelling causes more obstruction to air flow the smaller the child or infant.

The number of alveoli increases until age 10 to 12 years, but the number of bronchi do not increase after birth. Therefore, diseases which affect lung development can cause permanant ventilation perfusion mismatches if alveolar growth does not match that of the pulmonary vasculature development.

Males have smaller peripheral airways than females before school age, thus, pulmonary disease in male infants and children may be more severe than in females of the same age.

As soon as they can pick up objects, infants and toddlers are at risk for aspiration because they tend to put all small objects in their mouths.

Cardiac failure in infancy often presents as respiratory distress. Hepatomegaly in the infant with respiratory disrtess is the clue to congestive heart failure. It is confirmed by cardiomegaly on chest X-ray.

Cyanosis due to congenital right to left shunts does not improve with 100% oxygen inhalation; that due to respiratory disorders generally does.

Upper airway obstruction is usually manifest by inspiratory stridor and increased inspiratory effort (retractions); obstruction below the glottis is usually manifest by expiratory stridor, and may be accompanied by prolonged expiration and wheezing. If the child is not hoarse, the obstruction is likely subglottic or tracheal.

Oxygen difuses 20 times less readily across the capillary/alveolar surface than does carbon dioxide. Thus hypoxemia occurs relatively early in disorders of gas exchange and hypercapnia is a manifestation of a much more severe derangement of gas exchange.

Diagnostic modalities

Blood gas anaylsis

Arterial Blood Gasses

PaO_2 : values below 85 mm Hg breathing room air are abnormal, except in the very young infant. Respiratory failure is generally present when the value decreases to below 50 mm Hg.

$PaCO_2$: values above 45 mm Hg indicate hypoventilation, severe ventilation/perfusion mismatch or compenstation for chronic metabolic acidosis.

O_2 saturation: Because of the nature of the oxyhemoglobin dissociation curve, oxygen saturation does not decrease appreciably until arterial PO_2 decreases to about 60 torr (mm Hg)

Alveolar-arterial PO_2 difference

The PAO_2 - PaO_2 difference is a measurement of gas exchange which is not influenced by minute volume. Increases in the difference is indicative of shunts between the pulmonary and systemic circulations.

Alveolar PO_2 (PAO_2) can be estimated by the formula:

$$PAO_2 = FiO_2 \ (P_B - 47) - PaO_2/R$$

where

FiO_2 = inspired percent of oxygen

P_B = barometric pressure

R = carbon dioxide production/oxgyen consumption ratio: usually 0.8

Pulse oxymetery

A noninvasive method of monitoring O_2 saturation. It is affected by local vasoconstriction, however.

Radiography

Chest X-ray

A method for evaluation of structural aspects of the heart and lungs.

Lateral neck soft tissue X-ray

Useful for evaluation causes of upper airway obstruction. Penciling of the trachea is common in croup. The "thumb sign" is suggestive of epiglotitis. Soft tissue changes may be seen in retropharyngeal abscesses.

Contrast studies

Pulmonary arteriograms, bronchograms, thoracic aortograms, and barium swallows are sometimes useful in differentiating pulmonary problems.

Radioneuclide lung scans

These facilitate evaluation of pulmonary ventilation and perfusion.

Pulmonary Function Tests

In general, the child must be school age before he/she can cooperate sufficiently to perform these tests. When they can be done reliable, they are useful in identifying obstructive, restrictive or diffusion abnormalities. They are also helpful in quantating response to bronchodilators. The more commonly used pulmonary function tests are:

Spirometer
> Peak Expiratory Flow Rate (PEFR)
> Forced Vital Capacity (FEV)
> Forced Expiratory Volume in one second (FEV_1)
> FEV_1/FEV ratio

Pneumography
> One of the methods to assess neonatal apnea.

Flexible bronscopy
> Can be used with local anesthesia and thus in the ambulatory setting.

Rigid bronscopy
> Requires general sedation, but is necessary for foreign body removal.

Lung biopsy
> May be required for histologic or culture diagnosis. Can be done with needle aspiration.

Sweat Chloride
> Elevated in cystic fibrosis. False positive results are causes by Adrenal insufficiency, Malnutrition, Ectodermal dysplasia, Hypothyroidism, Nephrogenic diabetes insipidus, Mucopolysaccharidosis, Type I glycogen storage disease and Fucosidosis.

Pathophysiologic Manifestations

Symptoms
> Cough
>> A persistent cough is never normal in the neonate. A sudden onset of a paroxysmal cough should suggest foreign body aspiration.
>
> Sputum production
>> As a rule children swallow and hence "do not produce" sputum.
>
> Chest pain
>> The pain may be a clue to the location of pathology, but be aware of referred pain in evaluating the patient.
>
> Pleursy
>> Pain associated with and exacerbated by inspiration. It may be difficult to differentiate from chest wall pain in children, and can be a cause of splinting with respiration.

Physical Findings
> Respiratory Rate
>> Normal respiratory rates by age

Age	Breaths per minute
Newborn	30-60
Infant 1-6 months	30-40
Infant 6-12 months	24-30
1-4 years	20-30
4-6 years	20-25
6-12 years	16-20
Over 12 years	12-16

Grunting

An expiratory grunt is a compensatory mechanism for loss of lung volume. It is never a normal finding. It may indicate plerual involvement and is seen sometimes with intraabdominal problems such as peritiontis.

Flairing of the nasal alae

This is a sign of increased airway resistance.

Subcostal retractions

When small airway obstruction causes enough air trapping to depress the diaphragm, subcostal retractions will occur with inspiration.

Intercostal retractions

This is a reflection of inspiration against increased lung compliance.

Tracheal Deviation

May reflect a pneumothorax or atelectasis. Can be a clue to foreign body aspiration.

Cervical venous distention

Seen in conditions causing persistent increased intrathoracic pressure and in cardiac tamponade.

Stridor

Is indicative of upper airway obstruction.

Thoracic configuration

Chronic air trapping can produce a barrel chest configeration.

Breath Sounds

Normally the inspiration to expiration ratio is 2:1. this ratio is reversed in conditions resulting in bronchiolar obstruction.

Crackles/Rales

The term crackles is now preferred to rales. They are produced on inspiration by opening of small airways or alveoli.

Rhonchi/Wheezes

Expiratiory noises which are prolonged rather than discrete sounds. Wheezes are higher pitched and may be musical in quality.

Clubbing of nails

Most common pulmonary cause in children is cystic fibrosis.

Cyanosis

Cyanosis is the result of color changes due to the presence of at least 5 g of reduced Hb/dl. Central cyanosis is reflective of decreased oxygenation of the blood. It is due to a decreased oxygen saturation. Periphreal cyanosis is due to an increased arterial-venous oxygen difference and reflects local vascular stasis. The oxygen saturation is normal in periphreal cyanosis. Methemoglobin will produce cyanosis when it is exceeds more than 15% of the total hemoglobin.

Differential considerations in Apnea of Infancy

SIDS

CNS disorders
- Seizures
- Meningitis
- Encephalitis
- Intracranial hemorrhage (R/O shaken baby syndrome)
- Increased intracranial pressure
- Encephalopathy
- Central hypoventilation

Pulmonary disorders
- Pneumonia (especially RSV, pertussis)
- Pulmonary hemorrhage
- Pulmonary edema

Cardiovascular disorders
- Dysrhythmias
- Shock

Gastrointestinal disorders
- Gastroesophageal reflux
- Tracheoesophageal fistula
- Swallowing disorders

Metabolic disorders
- Hypoglycemia
- Hypocalcemia
- Hyponatremia
- Inborn Errors of Metabolism

Musculoskeletal disorders
- Infant botulism
- Guillian-Barre syndrome
- Congenital myopathies

Other
- Severe anemia
- Poisoning
- Hypothermia

Diagnostic considerations in Respiratory Distress

Upper Airway Disease
- Congenital causes
  - Vascular ring
  - Laryngeal web
  - Vocal cord paralysis
  - Laryngomalacia
  - Tracheomalacia
  - Micrognathia (Pierre Robin syndrome)
  - Glossoptosis (Down syndrome, Beckwith-Wiedmann syndrome, hypothyroidism)

- Infectious causes
  - Croup
  - Epiglottis
  - Bacterial trachitis
  - Peritonsillar abscess
  - Retropharyngeal abscess
  - Diphtheria

- Traumatic causes
  - Foreign body
  - Vocal cord paralysis
  - Subglottic stenosis
  - Scald burns to pharynx, epiglottis

- Allergic causes
  - Angioneurotic edema
  - Spasmodic croup

- Extrinsic masses/tumors

Lower Airway disease

- Congenital disorders
  - Cystic fibrosis
  - Emphsemia
  - Diagphramatic defects

- Infectious causes
  - Pneumonia
  - Bronchiolitis
  - Pleural effusions
  - Empyema

- Allergic disorders
  - Asthma
  - Anaphylaxis

- Cardiovascular disorders
  - Congestive heart failure
  - Pulmonary edema
  - Pulmonary embolism
  - Polycythemia
  - Severe anemia

- Traumatic causes
  - Bronchopulmonary dysplasia
  - Foreign body
  - Pneumothorax
  - Pulmonary contusion
  - Diaphragmatic defects
  - Near drowning
  - Spinal cord injury

- Neoplastic causes
  - Lung tumors
  - Mediastinal masses

- Other
  - Sarcoidosis
  - Musculoskeletal anomalies
  - Scolosis
  - Pulmanary hemosiderosis

Central Nervous System disease
- Infectious causes
  - Meningitis
  - Encephalitis

- Neuropathy/Myopathy causes
  - Guillian-Barre syndorme
  - Werdnig-Hoffmann syndrome
  - Muscular dystrophy
  - Myasthenia gravis
  - Infant botulism

- Other causes
  - Seizures
  - Poisonings

Metabolic disease
- Metabolic acidosis
  - Inborn Errors of Metabolism
  - Diabetes Mellitus
  - Sepsis
  - Dehydration
  - Salicylism
  - Other toxins

- Increased oxygen demand
  - fever
  - hyperthyroidism

Mediastinal Masses

Superior mediastinum
Cystic hygroma
Vascular tumors
Neurogenic tumors
Thymic tumors
Teratomas
Hemagnioma
Mediastinal abscess
Aortic aneuranism
Intrathracic thyroid
Esophageal lesion

Anterior Mediastimum
Thymoma
Thymic hyperplasia
Thymic cyst
Teratoma
Lymphoma
Vascular tumor
Intrathoracic thyroid
Pleuropericardial cyst
Lymphadenopathy

Posterior Mediastinum
Neurogenic tumors
Enterogenous cysts
Thoracic meningocele
Aortic aneurysm

Middle mediastinum
Lymphoma
Hypertrophic lymph nodes
Granuloma
Bronchogenic cyst
Enterogenic cysts
Metastasis
Pericardial cyst
Aortic anerysm
Anomalies of great vessels

In obstructive airway disease, such as asthma, a deceptive phase occurs during progression through more severe obstruction. At the severe stage, the child may become quieter because of tiring and evolving CO_2 narcosis, the wheezing may diminish because not enough air is moved to make the noise, and the pH and PCO_2 are normal. The next phase, however, is respiratory failure as depicted in the figure below:

Progression of pH and blood gas changes in asthma

Severity	pH	PaO$_2$	PaCO$_2$
Normal	7.40	98%	40 mmHg
Mild	mildly elevated	normal	mild decrease
Moderate	elevated	decrease	decrease
Severe	normal	marked decrease	normal
Respiratory Failrue	< 7.25	< 60 mmHg	> 60 mmHg

Disease Profiles

LARYNGOMALACIA
Alternate terminology
  infantile larynx
Etiology
  congenital anomaly
Pathophysiologic abnormality
  abnormally small and/or soft larynx
Symptoms
  stridor, especially with URI's
Laboratory findings
  Other: confirmed by bronchoscopy
Potential complications
  rarely may require tracheostomy
Differential diagnosis
  hypocalcemia, tracheal rings, neck and chest neoplasms
Therapeutic plan
  none usually needed
Prognosis
  good; stridor usually resolved by one year of age

BRONCHIOPULMONARY DYSPLASIA
Alternate terminology
BPD
Etiology
oxygen toxicity: $FiO_2 > 0.8$
barotrauma
Pathophysiologic abnormality
airway smooth muscle hypertrophy; interstitial edema from
endothelial injury
Predisposing conditions
oxygen and mechanical ventialtion treatment of
hyaline membrane disease
Physical findings
tachypnea, wheezing, crackles, retractions, cyanosis
Laboratory findings
Chest X-ray: characteristic fibrotic and cystic interstitial
changes in the chronic stage
ABG's: hypoxemia on room air
Potential complications
cor pulmonale, pulmonary hypertension
Therapeutic plan
Oxygen, diuretics, bronchodilators, calorie supplementation
Prognosis
may require oxygen supplimentation for a year after hospital
discharge, but may acquire normal pulmonary function by school
age; prone to HRAD.

CYSTIC FIBROSIS
Alternate terminology
mucoviscidosis
Etiology
autosomal recessive familial defect
Pathophysiologic abnormality
abnormal control of chloride channels in epithelial cells of
mucosal surfaces
Symptoms
failure to thrive, respiratory symptoms, chronic diarrhea,
intestinal maladsorption
Laboratory findings
sweat chloride > 60 mEq/L
Potential complications
recurrent pulmonary infections; malnutrition; hepatic cirrhosis
Therapeutic plan
aggressive treatment of pulmonary infections; pancreatic enzyme replacement
Prognosis
most now survive into adulthood

ASTHMA
Alternate terminology
Hyper Reactive Airway Disease (HRAD)
- a misnomer, but often used term
Pathophysiologic abnormality
Bronchospasm, Mucus production, mucosal edema
Predisposing conditions
Some, but not all are allergic in orgin; viral URI's often
trigger attacks
Symptoms
Cough (night cough, exercise induced cough are especially
characteristic), wheezing, dyspnea
Physical findings
Diffuse wheezing, signs of air trapping, use of accessory
muscles of respiration
Laboratory findings
Chest X-ray: hyperexpanded lung fields
ABG's: see chart above

Potential complications
  status asthmaticus, respiratory failure, pneumothorax
Differential diagnosis
  bronchiolitis, cystic fibrosis, tracheomaleacia, pertussis,
  foreign body aspiration, CHF
Therapeutic plan
  bronchodilators: theophylline, Beta-Adenergic
  anti-inflammatory agents: corticosteriods, Cromolyn

FOREIGN BODY ASPIRATION
 Pathophysiologic abnormality
  foreign body in trachea or bronchus
 Predisposing conditions
  access of small objects ot curious infants
 Symptoms
  sudden onset of cough, wheezing, respiratory distress
 Physical findings
  unilateral wheezing; deviation of trachea
 Laboratory findings
  Chest X-ray: mediastinal shift (toward lesion if atelectasis;
            away if ball valve obstruction)
 Differential diagnosis
  see asthma
 Therapeutic plan
  rigid bronchoscopy for removal

Jane E. Puls

Developmental Considerations

EARLY EMBRYONIC DEVELOPMENT

By the time an embryo has an ovulation age of 21 days the vascular system has began to appear as "blood islands", scattered masses of angiogenic cell clusters which increase in numbers and size, acquire a lumen and eventually form a vascular plexus. Part of the plexus differentiates in the main channels and at the cephalad end of the embryo these channels further specialize, producing a pair of heart tubes which come to lie parallel to each other and eventually fuse to form a single tube.

By 23 days of ovulation age differentiation continues into formation of the bulboventricular tube with an extra pericardial portion called the aortic sac. The cardiac loop forms and the caudal half of the bulboventricular tube begins to represent the early embryonic ventricle.

By an ovulation age of 25 days the heart completely occupies the pericardial cavity, with internally still a single tube but with primitive development of the left ventricle on the left side and the bulbos cordis on the right. A portion of the bulbos cordis eventually becomes the right ventricle.

Further development of the primitive atria and the truncus arteriosus occurs and by an ovulation age of about 27 days the external shape of the heart already suggests its future four chambered condition.

As the heart continues to develop, cardiac septation takes place, the ventricles enlarge in size, medial walls of the ventricles appose and fuse, forming the major portion of the muscular ventricular septum. The AV canal divides into a right and left atrioventricular orifice. Vascular structures change in their alignment and blood can begin to flow from one chamber to the other (an embryology text or specific book on the heart has further details on embryologic development).

As the heart continues development the pulmonary veins develop along with the atrioventricular valves. Septums continue formation, the chordae tendineae are initially formed, arterial valves are formed and the cardiovascular system increases in size and complexity.

Early in embryologic development aortic arches form (1st, 2nd, 3rd, 4th, and 6th, (the 5th aortic arch is generally not present in humans or is very rudimentary)). Aortic arches progress through a complex series of transformations. **The ductus arteriosus in the preborn child is the distal portion of the left 6th aortic arch. This obliterates after birth and is converted to the ligamentum arteriosum.**

Because the cardiovascular system in the fetus is required during fetal life for the supply of oxygenated blood to all tissues of the fetus, the cardiovascular system develops quite precociously. This results in complete organization of the cardiovascular system by an ovulation age of 8 weeks.

FETAL CIRCULATION

The fetal circulation has some marked differences from circulation in the post-born infant. Oxygenated blood is supplied to the fetal heart for distribution to the fetus from the placenta through the umbilical vein and has a PaO_2 of about 35mm Hg. Approximately 50% of this blood flows through the liver and the other 50% bypasses the liver through the ductus venosus into the inferior vena cava and to the right atrium. It then flows across the foramen ovale to the left atrium into the left ventricle, and is ejected into the ascending aorta from which is supplies the upper portion of the body. Blood returning through the superior vena cava flows through the right atrium and into the right ventricle, where it is ejected into the pulmonary arterial trunk. Most of this blood flows through the ductus arteriosus into the descending aorta and supplies the lower portion of the body. A portion of this blood will flow through the pulmonary arteries to the lungs.

Pulmonary resistance is much higher in the fetus than in the newborn and it accounts for blood preferentially crossing the ductus arteriosus and bypassing the lungs.

At birth fetal circulation stops and neonatal circulation begins. Changes that result in this include an initial fall in systemic blood pressure and then a progressive rise, a decrease in pulmonary vascular resistance with an increase in pulmonary blood flow, increased pulmonary venus return and left ventricular outflow, closure of the ductus arteriosus and the ductus venosus, and the formation of the ligamentum venosus and the ligamentum arteriosus. As well, the foramen ovale begins its apposition to the atrial wall and is functionally closed by 3 months of age.

Until the pulmonary vascular pressures decrease after birth to a level sufficiently below that of the systemic pressures, left to right flow will not occur through and the murmurs generated by such flow will not be heard.

Diagnostic Modalities

HISTORY - General history plus specific questioning about:
Cyanosis--resting
Blueness during exercise
Fatigue
Nocturnal dyspnea
Orthopnea
Failure to thrive or poor growth
Family history of congenital heart disease
Volume per feed
Dyspnic while sucking
Perspires profusely
Exhausted sleeping after feeds
Requires frequent feeds

PHYSICAL EXAMINATION:
Growth and development
Length average and weight decreased
Tachypnea
Liver enlargement
Spleen enlargement
Rales
Peripheral edema
Cyanosis
Clubbing
Cardiac rate - note normals for age:
Newborn 70 - 190
Infant 80 - 160
6 yrs. 75 - 115
10 yrs. 70 - 110
Adult   50 - 95
Character of the pulses
Blood pressure - varies by age
Normal (after 1 year of age) can be approximated by:
Systolic Blood Pressure = 80 + (age in years X 2)
Diastolic Blood Pressure = 2/3 of systolic pressure
Cardiac examination
Visual
Palpation
Auscultation

Physical Examination Findings suggestive of Heart Disease

Hepatomegaly	The neonate and infant rarely get pedal edema from CHF, but hepatomegaly is almost always present.
Cyanosis	3 to 5 g/dl of unsaturated Hgb is required to see cyanosis. Thus severe hypoxemia can be missed in patients who are anemic enough.
Precordial promenance	Reflective of long standing cardiomegaly during development of the chest wall.
Hyperdynamic precordium	Suggestive of extra volume load as in left to right shunts, if not in febrile children.
Any diastolic murmur	Diastolic murmurs should not be heard in normal healthy children.

Heart murmurs

Heart murmurs are classified according to their grade, location in the cardiac cycle, point of maximal intensity, the area of their radiation and the quality of their pitch.

Grades of Murmurs

Grade I	Soft heard only with difficulty
Grade II	Easily heard
Grade III	Loud but without a palpable thrill on the chest wall
Grade IV	Loud with a palpable thrill
Grade V	Heard with only one edge of the stethoscope on the chest
Grade VI	Heard without the stethoscope touching the chest

Cardiac cycle classification of murmurs

Systolic murmurs

Murmurs heard between the first heart sound (S_1) and the second heart sound (S_2).

Systolic ejection murmur (SEM)

There is a silent interval between S_1 and the onset of the murmur. It then crescendos to a maximum intensity and decrescendos to end before the S_2 heart sound. These murmurs arise in stenotic aortic or pulmonary valve areas and must overcome the pressure in such vessels before the flow rate is great enough to produce a murmur.

Holosystolic murmur

Also called pansystolic murmurs. These are the result of immediate flow from a high pressure area to a low flow area and are heard through out systole. Areas of such pressure differentials are from a ventricle to an atrium, or from the left ventricle to the right ventricle

End systolic murmur

Also called late systolic murmurs. These murmurs are caused by prolapse of the mitral valve toward the end of systole, allowing regurgitation of blood into the left atrium.

Diastolic murmurs

Murmurs heard between the second heart sound (S_2) and the first heart sound (S_1).

Early diastolic murmur

Murmurs beginning with S_2 are due to back flow through incompetent outflow tract valves and are generated by pressure in the aorta or pulmonary vessels. They rarely can be heard beyond mid diastole. Characteristically they are high pitched blowing murmurs.

Mid diastolic murmur

These murmurs are the result of turbulent flow over the mitral or tricuspid valves during the atrial filling phase of diastole. They are due to either an actual or relative (increased volume over normal sized valves) flow across these valves. These are usually very low pitched rumbling murmurs.

Late diastolic murmur

These are the result of end diastolic filling into a ventricle with decreased compliance, as occurs in ventricular hypertrophy. These may sound more like a click than a distinct murmur.

Continuous murmurs

Continuous murmurs continue through S_2. They begin in at least systole and continue in early diastole. A typical continuous murmur is that of a PDA. The systolic component is due to increased flow across a relatively stenotic pulmonary valve and the diastolic component is generated by the flow through the ductus from the aorta to the pulmonary vessel at the beginning of diastole.

Typical points of maximal intensity of murmurs

Aortic area: 2nd right intercostal space (ICS)
Pulmonary area: 2nd left intercostal space
Mitral area: the cardiac apex
Tricuspid area: left lower sternal border (LSB)

Typical qualities of murmurs

Blowing: high pitched.

This sound can be simulated by holding the stethoscope in the palm and stroking the back of the hand with the pad of a finger.

Harsh: medium pitched.

This sound can be simulated by holding the stethoscope in the palm and scratching the back of the hand with a fingernail.

Rumbling: low pitched.

This is the sound of a bowling ball rumbling down a gutter.

Characteristics of murmurs in selected heart lesions

Lesion	Loudest	Quality	Radiation
Aortic stenosis	Right 3rd ICS	Harsh, SEM	Carotids
Aortic regurgitation	MLSB	Blowing, Early diastolic	Apex
Pulmonary stenosis	Left 2nd ICS	Harsh, SEM	Lung fields
Pulmonary regurgitation	Left 2nd ICS	Low pitched, early-mid diast.	Little to none
Mitral stenosis	Apex	Low pitched, mid diast. rumble	None
Mitral regurgitation	Apex	Blowing, holosystolic	Left axilla
ASD	Left 2nd ICS	Harsh, SEM	Lung fields
VSD	LLSB	Harsh, holosystolic	None
PDA	Left 2nd-3rd ICS	Continuous	Lung fields

Characteristics of functional (Still's) murmurs

Systolic ejection murmur
Grade III or less
Vibratory quality
Non radiating

CHEST X-RAY - Note size of heart and amount of pulmonary blood flow (heart size normally occupies 50% or less of the chest and pulmonary vessels are seen from the hyler area throughout 2/3 of the chest)

ELECTROCARDIOGRAM - Shows malcardio mass as it is reflected by electrical activity seen at the surface and shows cardiac rythmn.

As a result of fetal circulation, the newborn heart has a relative right ventricular hypertrophy. The muscle mass of the right ventricle is roughly equal to the mass of the left ventricle. Postnatal the left ventricular muscle mass begins to increase and gradually irrelative right ventricular hypertrophy resolves.

Most children's heart disease is "structural" rather than the "functional" heart disease seen in adults. Children's hearts are generally, if you will, "malformed" rather than "malfunctioning". These diseases are reflected in different ways in the electrocardiogram (see under disease profiles).

ECHOCARDIOGRAPHY - Forms available now include immode and two dimensional echocardiography, as well as, pulsed continuous wave and color flow doppler. These forms now give precise information about cardiac structure and blood flow and essential adjunct in evaluation of the patient **when done by an experienced echocardiographer with interpretation by a pediatric cardiologist.**

Echocardiography is and incredibly versatile tool for prenatal diagnosis of both structural and functional congenital heart disease. It should be routinely included as a part of the prenatal ultrasound.

EXERCISE TESTING - Used most commonly in patients with known heart disease to assess effective exercise on cardiac function, as a guide to prescribing activity for the child.

Most helpful in children with:
Arrhythmias
Chronic volume overload of the ventricles
Left ventricular outflow obstruction
Hypertension

RADIONUCLIDE STUDIES - A relatively non-invasive procedure that can be used to assess blood flow, shunts, etc. Can even be used on a portable basis. Does not provide the information about anatomic details provided by echocardiography and catheterization but may be useful in some patients.

CARDIAC CATHETERIZATION - Always a good tool for delineation of anatomy and understanding of directional flow in an individual's heart, the cardiac cath is used less frequently since the advent of echocardiography. However, it remains a good tool for this purpose and essential tool for the measurement of PaO_2, etc. in the various chambers of the heart. This information is considered necessary for planning corrective surgery, etc. for a child.

LABORATORY DATA - Some or all of these may be appropriate depending on the patients particular situation. Patients who are polycythemic as a result of their heart disease frequently have other hematologic abnormalities.

Arterial blood gas
Serum chemistries
Complete blood count
Frequent follow-up of hemoglobin and hematocrit
Platelet count
Fibrinogen level
PT/PTT

Pathophysiologic Manifestations

Supraventricular tachycardia in the neonate and infant is often initially mistakenly diagnosed as sepsis.

Only 40 - 50% of CHD (Congenital Heart Disease) is diagnosed by one week of age. Only 50 - 60% of CHD is diagnosed by one month of age.

Incidence of CHD is 10 times higher in still born than in live born infants.

Incidence of CHD in still borns, plus spontaneous abortions, plus live borns, is five times that of the incidence of CHD in live borns alone.

Incidence in the live born child of CHD is approximately 1% (varies from .4 - 1.0 depending on the study.) this number is probably an under estimation.

It is felt that most estimates under represent CHD because the majority of the studies that estimates are based on were done when Echo was not available, and some things (like bicuspid aortic valve, occurs in approximately 2% of the population) are best diagnosed with Echo.

Risk for recurrence - this is impossible to predict in the overall since, partly because it is different for specific lesions. In general, the recurrence risk is higher if the proband has a more serious lesion, if the affected parent is the mother, or if more than one first degree relative is affected. Recurrence risk for siblings is approximately 2 - 3%. Transmission risk to next generation is approximately 5 - 10%.

Common chromosomal abnormalities associated with CHD (chromosomal defects account for 5 - 8% of CHD).

Single gene defects - account for 3% of CHD.
    Autosomal dominant:
                Marfan's - aortic and mitral valve incompetence, dilatation of the
                        ascending aorta.
                Holt - Oram - VSD, ASD
                Noonan's - PSASD cardio myopathy
    Autosomal recessive:
                Pompe's (Type II A glycogen storage disease) -cardio myopathy.
                Ellis - VanCreveld - AVSD, common atrium
    X linked:
                Duchuenne Muscular Dystrophy - cardio myopathy

Polygenic inheritance.
        Well described for PDA with a recurrence risk of 2.5% in siblings
        (recurrence risk increased to 10% if > than one family member affected).

Some CHD's are more common in one sex than the other:
        AS - more common in males
        Coarctation - more common in males
        ASD - more common in females
        PDA - more common in females
        VSD - equal in both sexes

The most common form of CHD is VSD (30 - 40% of all CHD).

Congenital syndromes associated with Congenital Heart Disease

Syndrome	Heart lesion
Trisomy 13	VSD, ASD, PDA
Trisomy 18	VSD, ASD, PDA
Trisomy 21	Endocardial cushion defect
Turner syndrome	Coaractation of the aorta, aortic stenosis
Williams syndrome	supravalvular aortic stenosis
Noonan syndrome	Pulmonary valve stenosis, aortic valve stenosis
Holt-Oram syndrome	ASD, VSD
Marfan syndrome	Mitral valve prolapse, aortic valve regurgitation, dilated and dissecting aorta
Asplenia syndrome	Complex cyanotic hearl lesions, anomalous pulmonary venous return, dextrocardia, single ventricle, single AV valve
Polysplenia syndrome	Pulmonary atresia, dextrocardia, single ventricle, azygos continuation of inferior vena cava
Congenital rubella	PDA, peripheral pulmonic stenosis
Glycogen storage disease	Hypertrophic cardiomyopathy
DiGeorge syndrome	Aortic arch anomalies, tetralogy of Fallot, pulmonary atresia, transposition of great vessels, truncus arteriosis

CHARGE association
  Coloboma
  Heart lesion
  Atresia of choanae
  Retardation
  Genital anomalies
  Ear anomalies
	Tetralogy of Fallot, endocardial cushion defects, VSD, ASD

VATER association
  Vertebral anomalies
  Anal anomalies
  Tracheo-
  Esophageal anomalies
  Radial and renal anomalies
	VSD

Common causes of heart failure by age

Fetus

      Severe anemia

      Supraventricular tachycardia

      Ventricular tachycardia

      Complete block

premature infant

      Cardiomyopathy from: asphyxia, sepsis, hypoglycemia, hyopcalcemia

      Fluid overload

      PDA

      VSD

      Cor Pulmonale from BPD

Term infant

      Cardiomyopathy from: asphyxia, sepsis, hypoglycemia, hyopcalcemia

      A-V malformation (vein of Galen, Hepatic)

      Left-sided obstructrive lesions (hypoplastic left heart, Coaractation of aorta)

      Large mixing cardiac defects (single ventricle, truncus arteriosus)

      Viral myocarditis

Infant-Toddler

      Left to right cardiac shunts (VSD)

      Hemangioma (arteriovenous malformation)

      Anomalous left coronary artery

      Metabolic cardiomyopathy

      Acute hypertension (hemolytic-uremic syndrome)

      Supraventricular tachycardia

      Kawasake disease

Child-Adolescent

      Rheumatic fever

      Acute hypertension

      Viral myocarditis

      Thyrotoxicosis

      Hemochromatosis-hemosiderosis

      Cancer therapy (radiation, adriamycin)

      Sickle cell anemia

      Endocarditis

      Cor pulmonale (cystic fibrosis)

      Status asthmaticus

Acyatotic Congenital Heart Lesions

With increased pulmonary blood flow (vascularity) [left to right shunts]
    Atrial Septal Defect
    Patent Ductus Arteriosis
    Ventricular Septal Defect
    Endocardial Cushion Defect
    Arteriovenous Malformation

With normal pulmonary blood flow [no left to right shunt]
    Coaraction of the aorta
    Aortic Stenosis
    Pulmonary Stenosis
    Mitral Stenosis
    Mitral regurgitation
    Endocardial fibroelastosis

Cyanotic Congenital Heart Lesions

With decreased pulmonary flow (vascularity) [pulmonary outflow obstruction]
    Pulmanary stenosis
    Pulmonary atresia
    Tetralogy of Fallot
    Tricuspid atresia
    Pulmonary atresia and hypoplastic right ventricle
    Ebstein anomaly

With increased pulmonary blood flow [right to left shunt]
    Hypoplastic left heart syndrome
    Total anomalous pulmonary venous return
    Transposition of great vessels
    Single ventricle complexes
    Truncus arteriosus

Therapeutic Considerations

Lesions amenable to Prostaglandin (PGE$_1$) palliation

Hypoplastic left-heart syndrome
Complex coarctation syndromes
Critical aortic stenosis
Hypoplastic right-heart syndromes
     Pulmonary atresia with intact ventricular septum
     Tricuspid atresia
Pulmonary atresia with VSD

Mneumonic for treating CHF/pulmonary edema

		Mechanism of action
U	Upright position	Improve ventilation-perfusion
N	Nifedipine, nitroglycerine, nitroprusside	Afterload reduction
L	Lasix	Diuresis, fluid shift
O	Oxygen	Improved O$_2$ saturation
A	Albuterol inhalation	Bronchodilation
D	Dopamine, dobutamine, digitalis	Inotropic agents
M	Morphine	Anxiolytic, venous pooling
E	Extremety tourniquets	Decrease preload

Surgical procedures for selected CHD lesions

Pallitive procedures

Procedure	Anatomy involved	Result	Indicated for
Blalock-Taussig shunt	Subclavian artery to ipsilateral pulmonary artery	Increased pulmonary blood flow	Tetralogy of Fallot pulmonary valve atresia
Waterston shunt	aorta to right pulmonary artery	Increased pulmonary blood flow	Tetralogy of Fallot pulmonary valve atresia tricuspid atresia
Rashkind procedure	balloon aria septostomy	Increased atrial mixing	transposition of great arteries tricuspid atresia
Blalock-Hanlon procedure	operative atrial septostomy	Increased atrial mixing	transposition of great arteries
Balloon angioplasty	valves and vessels	dilation of valves/vessels	pulmonary valve stenosis aortic valve stenosis
Pulmanary artery banding	pulmonary artery	decreased pulmonary blood flow	VSD endocardial cushing defect single ventricle

Corrective procedures

Procedure	Anatomy involved	Result	Indicated for
Fontan procedure	right atrium to pulmonary artery anastomosis	atrium functions as right ventricle	tricuspid atresia single ventricle pulmonary atresia
Mustard procedure	intra-atrial baffle	RV remains systemic ventricle	transposition of great arteries
Norwood procedure	a complex two stage procedure		hypoplastic left heart

Disease Profiles

PERSISTENT FETAL CIRCULATION

Not necessarily classified as a congenital heart disease, but typically occurs in the newly born full term infant. Presents much like Cyanotic Congenital Heart Disease.

Alternate Terminology:
PFC

Etiology:
Uncertain in some cases, but most commonly related to perinatal hypoxemia.

Pathophysiology:
Generally persistent pulmonary hypertension which results in left to right shunting through the foramen ovale and/or the patent ductus arteriosus.

Predisposing Conditions:
Hypoxic insult at birth.

Symptoms:
Tachypnea in the first few hours of life with varying degrees of respiratory distress.

Physical Examination:
Ill appearance, +/- systolic murmur, +/- a loud second heart sound, +/- perasternal heave.

Laboratory Findings:
Acidosis, x-ray with decreased vascular flow, echo with right to left flow seen at the foramen ovale.

Differential Diagnosis:
Includes the Cyanotic Congenital Heart Diseases, most specifically transposition of the great arteries.

Potential Complications:
Almost universally fatal if not treated, and even when treated has significant mortality.

Diagnostic Plan:
Diagnosis based on physical exam plus x-ray, greatly helped by echocardiography and measurement of differential PaO_2's.

Therapeutic Plan:
Oxygen administration, mechanical ventilation, correction of acidosis and any electrolyte abnormalities, administration of Tolazoline and consideration of possible use of ECMO (Extra Corporeal Membrane Oxygenation).

Congenital Structural Lesions

HYPOPLASTIC LEFT-HEART SYNDROME

Pathophysiologic abnormality
Underdevelopment of the aortic root, aortic valve, left ventricle or mitral valve. Either or both valves may be atretic. Systemic flow is duct dependent.

Predisposing conditions

Symptoms
Severe CHF and cardiovascular collapse occur as the duct closes.

Physical findings
Signs of poor periphreal perfusion (mottling of skin, prolonged capillary refill, deminished or absent pulses) and congestive failure. A nonspecific murmur may be present.

Laboratory findings
X-ray: cardiomegaly, pulmonary congestion

EKG: normal for age
ECHO: is diagnositc

Chronologic sequence of manifestations
Failure occurs early as the duct begins to close in the first few days or weeks of life

Differential diagnosis
Critical aortic stenosis, severe coarctation of aorta

Theraputic plan
Prostaglandin E1, supportive care
Norwood procedure may allow survial through infancy

HYPOPLASTIC RIGHT-HEART SYNDROME

Alternate terminology
Either of the following can causethis syndorme:
Pulmonary atresia with intact ventricular septum
Tricuspid atresia with a patent ASD

Pathophysiologic abnormality
Pulmonary perfusion is dependent on a patent ductus arteriosis in pulmonary atresia

Predisposing conditions

Symptoms
Severe cyanosis at birth

Physical findings
A continuous PDA murmur may be heard in the pulmonary atresia defect

Laboratory findings
Chest X-ray: diminished pulmonary vascularity; variable heart size
EKG: right atrial enlargement; left axis deviation in tricuspid atresia
Echo: is diagnostic

Chronologic sequence of manifestations
Rapid deterioratin\on as the ductus closes

Differential diagnosis
Severe pulmonary stenosis, Tetratology of Fallot

Theraputic plan
Prostaglandin E1, supportive care
Surgical establishment of a aortico-pulmonary artery shunt

ATRIAL SEPTAL DEFECT

The most common CHD found in <u>adults</u> (discounting congenital bicuspid aortic valve).

Alternate Terminology:
ASD, Ostium Primum (Defect Ostium   Secundum (Defect at the Fossa Ovalis)).

Predisposing conditions:
More common in female, with 2 to 1 ratio, female to male. Genetics multifactorial, but some Mendelian examples available.

Symptoms:
Usually asymptomatic, may have mild fatigue. If persists uncorrected into adulthood, may develop fatigue, dyspnea, chest pain, etc.

Physical Findings:
Growth and development usually normal, +/-right ventricular systolic lift, +/- accentuated first heart sound, plus fixed splitting of second heart sound, plus systolic murmur at LUSB.

Laboratory Findings:
CXR - Some heart enlargement, prominence of pulmonary vasculature.
EKG - Regular sinus rhythm pattern.
ECHO - Show left to right shunt with resultant right sided volume overload. Sometimes (usually) can visualize and categorize actual defect.
Cath - Increased O_2 saturation in right side of heart.

Chronologic Sequence of Manifestations:
Few findings early in life, so many individuals not diagnosed until adulthood. As adults, may develop pulmonary hypertension and congestive heart failure or atrial arrhythmias.

Differential Diagnosis:
Valvular - competent foramen ovale.

Potential Complications:
Pulmonary Hypertension, congestive heart failure, atrial fibrillation or flutter, mitral valve prolapse, infections.

Diagnositc Plan:
Usually murmur noted on routine exam leads to chest x-ray, EKG, ECHO, and possibly Catheter.

Therapeutic Plan:
Watchful waiting in younger children with elective repair prior to school age. Repair adults. Repair is usually direct repair or patch repair of defect. Genetic counseling about inheritance.

VENTRICULAR SEPTAL DEFECT

Very common. Occurs as an isolated defect in > 20% of all CHD and in conjunction with other defects in > 25% of CHD.

Alternate Terminology:
VSD

Etiology:
Prenatal incomplete development of the ventricular septum.

Pathophysiology:
Depends on the size of the defect. Small defects have high resistance to flow across the defect, with little resultant shunting. Moderate defects have significant left to right shunting, with much higher pressures in the left ventricle than the right. Large defects have relatively complete mixing of the blood in the ventricles, with right ventricular pressure equal to left.

Symptoms:
Depends on the size of the defect. Small - asymptomatic. Large - congestive failure symptoms (sweating, tachypnea, grunting respirations, fatigue with feeds).

Physical Findings:
Systolic murmur, +/- LLSB thrill. Child with large defects have respiratory distress, decreased weight for height, narrowly split S^2, hepatomegaly.

Laboratory Findings:
CXR - Small defect - normal. Large defect - enlarged heart with prominent pulmonary vascular markings.
EKG - Large defect - QRS axis oriented to the right, bilaterally increased ventricular voltage, increased left atrial voltage.
Echo - Images defect. Invaluable.
Cath - Reflection of left to right shunt found in increased O_2 saturation of blood in right ventricle.

Chronologic sequence of manifestations:
Most small isolated VSD's are insignificant and close spontaneously. Large VSD's +/- other defects progress to congestive failure with pulmonary damage.

Diagnostic Plan:
Diagnosis based on physical exam plus x-ray and ECHO. ECHO demonstrates not only size and location of defect, but blood flow across defect.

Therapeutic Plan:
Surgical repair of moderate or large defects. Most small defects are followed with repeat exams and close spontaneously.

ATRIOVENTRICULAR CANAL DEFECT

Atrioventricular Canals are generally described in two basic types:
Partial (comprised of ostium primum Atrial Septal Defect, cleft mitral valve and deficient ventricular septum, but without significant interventricular shunting)
Complete (Atrial Septal Defect, essentially single valve from atria to ventricles comprised of tissue of mitral and tricuspid valves, and deficient ventricular septum with shunting.
Complete form much less common and much more severe than partial form. About half of children with Down's Syndrome have Congenital Heart Disease, and a large percentage of this is the Atrioventricular Canal.

Alternate Terminology:
AV Canal, Endocardial Cushion Defect

Etiolgy:
Incomplete growth of the endocardial cushions.

Pathophysiology:
Atrial Septal Defect of the lower part of the septum, cleft mitral valve +/- cleft tricuspid valve and inadequate tissue of the ventricular septum.

Associated conditions:
Nearly all patients with Asplenia Syndrome have a complete Atrioventricular Canal. Other associated conditions include: Tetralogy of Fallot, polysplenia, disorder of right ventricle, Down's Syndrome.

Symptoms:
Depends on type: Partial have symptoms similar to patients with simple Atrial Septal Defect unless their mitral valve is compromised to the point that they have significant mitral regurg. Then they are likely to have fatigue, dyspnea, failure to gain weight adequately, repeated respiratory infections, etc. Those with complete Atrioventricular Canals progress rapidly to congestive heart failure and generally do very poorly without corrective surgery.

Physical Findings:
Partial: +/- systolic murmur at LVSB, +/-holosystolic blowing, murmur at the apex. Complete: plus systolic murmur at LVSB, plus systolic murmur at LLSB, plus fixed splitting of second heart sound, +/- hepatomegaly and evidence of congestive heart failure.

Laboratory Findings:
CXR - Cardiac enlargement +/- pulmonary congestion
EKG - Superior orientation of the mean QRS axis in the frontal plane, +/- prolonged QT interval.
ECHO - Visualization of Atrial Septal Defect, valvular function, Ventricular Septal Defect with evaluation of shunt, and evaluation of ventricular size and ability that may influence surgical plans.
Cath - Increased O_2 saturation in right atrium, increased right ventricular pressure (in complete type).

Chronologic sequence of manifestations:
Partial defects progress as Atrial Septal Defects with an increased risk of infection 2° to mitral valve deformity. Complete defects usually progress rapidly to congestive heart failure and die if not corrected in some fashion.

Differential Diagnosis:
Must distinguish from simple Atrial Septal Defect, simple Ventricular Septal Defect, and must delineate type.

Potential Complications:
High risk of endocardial infection with valvular disease, many children (especially with complete Atrioventricular

Canal) have associated disease.

Diagnostic Plan:
Diagnose with high level of suspicion (Asplenia Syndrome, Down's Syndrome), history, physical, especially EKG and ECHO.

Therapeutic Plan:
Medical management in those with fewer symptoms, surgical correction in those with significant mitral regurg or complete Atrioventricular Canal. Small infants may require pulmonary banding (to decrease pressure to lung fields) until at an age where surgical correction if possible.

PATENT DUCTUS ARTERIOSUS
Alternate terminology
PDA
Etiology
Failure of the ductus arteriosus to close after birth
Pathology
Pathogenesis
Pathophysiologic abnormality
The direction of flow through the duct is dependent on the relative pressures in the systemic and pulmonary circuits, it can be either left-to right or visa versa
Predisposing conditions
prematurity
Symptoms
Large left-to-right shunts can result in failure to thrive, CHF; right-to-left shunts cause dyspnea and cyanosis
Physical findings
Bounding pulses are characteristic of large left-to-right shunts
A continuous murmur is present after the pulmonary pressure decreases enough for a large shunt ot occur
Laboratory findings
Chest X-ray: cardiomegaly and increased pulmonary vascularity in large left-to-right shunts
EKG: biventricular hypertrophy; right ventricular hypertrophy indicates development of increased pulmonary resistence
Potential complications
Pulmonary hypertension
Theraputic plan
Surgical ligation of the duct before pulmonary hypertension develops
Prognosis
Good if corrected. If pulmonary hypertension develops (usually after a year), it is irreversible

CONGENITAL MITRAL STENOSIS
Commonly associated with PDA, AS, coarc.
Etiology:
Malformed male valve, funnel-shaped, with thickened leaflets and short, deformed cordae tendineae.
Symptoms:
Underdeveloped infants with dyspnea 2^0 to CHF. Cyanosis. Pallor.
Physical Findings:
Rumbling diastolic murmur followed by a loud first sound. Second sound split and loud.
Laboratory Findings:
EKG - RVH
X-ray - Left atrial and right ventricular enlargement, pulmonary congestion.
Echo - Enlarged left atrium, thick mitral valve leaflets.
Cath - Increased pressure in right ventricle, posterior, anterior and pulse capillaries.

Therapeutic Plan:
Poor prognosis. Mitral valve prothesis. Usually die early.

AORTIC STENOSIS
Etiology
Congenital (usually bicuspid); acquired in Rheumatic fever; or part of Williams syndrome
Pathophysiologic abnormality
Outflow obstruction to the left ventricle
Symptoms
most patients are asymptomatic until adulthood when syncope, easy fatigibliety or anginal pain may occur
Physical findings
Harsh systolic ejection murmur at right 2nd ICS, radiating to caroids; systolic thrill at jugular notch
Laboratory findings
Chest X-ray: Post stenotic dilitation of aorta
EKG: left ventricular hypertrophy
Echo: identifies the lesion and location
Theraputic plan
Bacterial endocarditis prophylaxis;
Surgical repair if severity warrants

COARCTATION OF THE AORTA
Etiology
Pathology
Pathogenesis
Pathophysiologic abnormality
Predisposing conditions
male sex or Turner syndrome in females
Symptoms
rarely: fatigue, leg cramps, headaches
Physical findings
Small shoe size for age may be a clue; deminished femoral pulses; hypertension (in arms) if long standing
Laboratory findings
Chest X-ray: rib notching (> 5 years old); abnormal aortic knob
EKG: may show LVH if severe and prolonged
Echo: sometimes can visualize the lesion
Chronologic sequence of manifestations
About 10% develop CHF in infancy
Theraputic plan
Bacterial endocarditis prophylaxis is indicated;
Surgical repair

PULMONARY STENOSIS
Pathophysiologic abnormality
cyanosis results from decreased pulmonary perfusion, and in severe stenosis with increased right atrial pressure, from a right-to-left shunt through the foramen ovale Periphreal pulmonary stenosis is a different lesion associated with congenital rubella syndrome
Symptoms
most are asymptomatic
Physical findings
cyanosis,if severe; systolic ejection murmur at 2nd left ICS radiating into posterior lung fields
Laboratory findings
Chest X-ray: decreased pulmonary vascularity and cardiomegaly if the stenosis is severe
EKG: degree of right axis deviation correlates with severity of stenosis

Theraputic plan
Bacterial endocarditis prophylaxis
Surgical repair or balloon angioplaxis if severity
warrants

TETRALOGY OF FALLOT
Most common cyanotic congenital heart lesion
Pathophysiologic abnormality
1. right ventricular outflow obstruction (pulmonary stenosis)
2. Dextroposition of aorta (overrides the ventricular septum
3. Ventricular septal defect
4. Right ventricular hypertrophy
The degree of right ventricular outflow obstruction
govern the degree of hypoxemia and right-to-left shunt
Physical findings
cyanosis; harsh holosystolic murmur at LSB; squatting
posture; exertional dyspnea
Laboratory findings
Chest X-ray: Boot shaped normal size heart;
decreased pulmonary vascularity; may have
right sided aortic arch
EKG: right axis deviation, RVH
Echo: is diagnositc
Potential complications
Hypercyanotic spells (Tet spells)
Theraputic plan
Bacterial endocarditis prophylaxis
Surgical pallatiation: Blalock-Taussig procedure
Definifitive surgical repair

PERSISTENT TRUNCUS ARTERIOSUS
Pathophysiologic abnormality
Single trunk from the heart; pulmonary arteries arise
from this trunk; a large VSD is present
Symptoms
Physical findings
Findings relate to size of pulmonary artery and may
resemble either a PDA or Tetrology of Fallot
Laboratory findings
Echo: is diagnostic
Theraputic plan
Surgical repair may be done

D-TRANSPOSITION OF THE GREAT ARTERIES
Alternate terminology
simple transposition of the great vessels
Pathophysiologic abnormality
pulmonary and systemic blood are recirculated through
their own circuits; a communication between the
circuits (ASD, VSD, PDA) must exist for survival
Predisposing conditions
more common in males
Physical findings
cyanosis is present at birth
Laboratory findings
Chest X-ray: egg-on-a-string appearance of heart
Chronologic sequence of manifestations
CHF develops early if surgical communication between
the two circuits is not created
Theraputic plan
Balloon atrial septostomy (Rashkin procedure) may be
lifesaving; an atrial switch procedure can be done later

L-TRANSPOSITION OF THE GREAT ARTERIES
Alternate terminology
corrected transposition of the great vessels
Pathophysiologic abnormality

there are usually associated anomalies which
determine the exact nature of this complex lesion for
any individual patient

TOTAL ANOMALOUS VENOUS RETURN
Alternate terminology
TAPVR
Etiology
Pathology
Pathogenesis
Pathophysiologic abnormality
pulmonary venous return is not to the left atrium but
instead to one or a combination of the following routes:
Supracardiac (into the innominate vein)
Cardiac (into the coronary sinus or back to the right atrium)
Infracardiac (infradiaphragmatic-into the inferior vena cava)
Each of these lesions must have a right-to-left shunt,
usually via the foramen ovale; pulmonary venous
obstruction is often present and its degree determines
the degree of cyanosis present
Laboratory Findings:
Chest X-ray: typical "snowman" or figure 8 heart shape
Theraputic plan
Surgical reimplantation of the veins into the left atrium

PARTIAL ANOMALOUS PULMONARY VENOUS RETURN
Alternate Terminology:
PAPVR
PATHOPHYSIOLOGY:
One or more of the pulmonary veins returns to the right
atrium instead of to the left atrium, sometimes
associated with an Atrial Septal Defect.
SYMPTOMS:
Depends on number of veins with anomalous
connection. Single vein, usually asymptomatic.
Multiple veins, symptoms of fatigue and dyspnea.
PHYSICAL FINDINGS:
+/- right ventricular systolic lift, plus widely split (but not
fixed splitting) of second heart sound.
LABORATORY FINDINGS:
CXR - Some enlargement of right side of heart,
increased pulmonary vasculature.
EKG - +/- evidence of right volume overload.
ECHO - Plus increase right-sided flow seen, +/
visualization of anomalous vein(s).
Cath - May be able to directly enter anomalous veins and
visualize return with contrast.
CHRONOLOGIC SEQUENCE OF MANIFESTATIONS:
Depends on number of anomalous veins. Increased
return to right side of heart leads to congestive heart
failure.
THERAPEUTIC PLAN:
In patients with large right-sided return, large left to right
shunts through associated Atrial Septal Defects or
pulmonary hypertension with congestive heart failure,
surgical correction is required.

Acquired Structural Lesions

KAWASAKI DISEASE
Pathophysiologic abnormality
characterized by coronary aneurysms

Jill E. Adler

Developmental Considerations

Hematopoiesis is the physiologic system whereby the human body produces distinct blood cell lines. The primary organs involved in this process are the bone marrow, liver, spleen, thymus and lymph nodes.

Formation of hematopoietic elements takes place in the human embryo yolk sac by the third week post conception. By division and differentiation, stem cells give rise to committed progenitor cells which are the precursors of erythroid and myeloid cell lines.

Active hematopoiesis occurs by two months of fetal life, and is initially centered in the liver, shifting to the bone marrow by 6 months gestational age. At birth, most hematopoiesis takes place in the bone marrow.

In infants, the medullary spaces of most bones contain hematopoietic tissue, but as childhood progresses, the marrow in long bones is replaced by fatty tissue. Cells in the skull, clavicles, scapulaes, sternum, ribs, vertegrae and pelvis are responsible for the production of most hematopoetic elements in older children and adults. However, if significant loss of blood cells occurs, the long bone morrow can reactivate and produce blood.

The hormone which regulates the rate of division and differentiation of red blood cells is erythropoeitin. Its prohormone is produced by the renal glomerulus primarily in response to tissue hypoxia, and activation occurs within serum. Interleukin-3 and OM-CFS are factors dependent on erythropoetin which stimulate progenitors. The newborn infant is relatively polycythcmic since low intrauterine PO_2 levels stimulate erythropoetin production. PaO_2 rises after birth, activating an inhibitory feedback loop which decreases erythropoetin productions. The infant becomes relatively anemic until erythropoeitin production is again stimulated by the declining red cell population. By 3 to 4 months post birth, erythropoetin levels have risen and subsequently serve to maintain red blood cell hemostasis.

Approximately ninety percent of the dry weight of the mature red cell is made up of hemoglobin, the oxygen carrying protein. In the fetus, at 6 months, 90% of the hemoglobin is hgbF. It contains gamma polypepticle chains in place of the beta chains of hgbA. At birth, 70% of total hemoglobin is F, and it decreases rapidly therafter, to less than 2% of the total hemaglobin by 6 to 12 months of age.

The mature red cell, because its nucleus has been lost, has a finite life span of approximately 120 days. The red cell of a newborn infant has a life span of approximately 90 days. It has no mitochondria, so glucose is primarily utilized by anaerobic glycolysis.

Lymphoid and myeloid elements derive from the same pluripotent stem cell as erythrocytes and megakaryocytes. The first stage of differentiation forms a lymphoid stem cell which elaborates T, B and plasma cells, and a trilineage myeloid stem cell which produces erythrocytes, megakaryocytes, polymorphonuclear leukocytes, monocyte-maerophages and eosinophils.

Polymorphonuclear leukocytes, or neutrophils are the predominant granulocyte and have ameoboid motility, are chemotactic and can actively phagocytize. Serum neutrophils consist of a circulating pool and a marginal pool of neutrophils sequestered in small blood vessels. After circulating for an average of 6 to 9 hours, they enter the tissue to carry out their primary function of phagocytosis.

Eosinophils normally comprise less than 5% of circulating leukocytes. Their concentration may be increased during convalescence from viral infections, in association with Hodkins disease, parasitic and allergic disorders and familial hyperesinophilia.

Basophils contain large amounts of heparin and histamine, and comprise less than 1% of circulating lymphocytes. Increased basophil counts may be seen in mastocytosis and chronic mycoglobulous leukemia.

Lymphocytes are motile cells, but do not perform phagocytosis. They can be characterized on the basis of physical and immunological components as T or B cells. A relative lymphocytosis can be seen with pertussis, viral infections and infectious lympocytosis. Atypical lymphocytes are characteristic of Epstein-Barr virus infection.

Monocytes are phagocytic cells which comprise 1 to 5% of circulating leukocytes. Increases in monocyte levels are noted with tuberculosis, systemic mycosis, bacterial endocarditis and some protozoan infections. When monocytes enter tissues they become macrophagics and hepatic kupfer cells.

Diagnostic Modalities

Complete Blood Count (CBC)
 Hgb (hemoglobin) - concentration
 Hct (hematocrit) - packed cell volume
 RBC - red blood cell count
 RBC indexes
  MCV (Mean Cell Volume) - average volume of red cells
  MCH (Mean Cell Hemoglobin) - weight of Hgb of the average red cell
  MCHC (Mean Cell Hemoglobin Concentration) - average concentration of
   hemoglobin in a given volume of packed red cells
 WBC - Leukocyte count
 WBC differential - percentage of different components of the total white blood cell count

Reticulocyte Count - the number of nucleated RBC's in the periphreal smear; it reflects the
 bone marrow's capability to respond to a fall in peripheral red blood cell numbers.

Peripheral Smear - sample of peripheral blood is placed on a slide & fixed with Wright's stain. Manual
 observation is used to determine staining quality and morphology of blood components.

Iron Studies
 Serum iron
 Serum ferritin
 Erythrocyte porphyrins
 Total iron binding capacity (TIBC)
 Percent saturation of TIBC

Hemoglobin Electrophoresis - measures concentrations of hemoglobin variants.

Bone Marrow Aspirate and Biopsy - tissue samples obtained from sternum, anterior or posterior iliac
 crests, tibia or vertebral spinous process which allow assessment of cellularity, distribution and
 maturation of cells and presence of rare or abnormal cells.

Erythrocyte Osmotic Fragility Test - indicates shape change of the red blood cell from the normal biconcave disc. Helps establish diagnosis of hereditary spherocytosis.

Pathophysiologic considerations

Anemia

Anemia can be diagnosed when red cell volume of hemoglobin falls two standard deviations below that of the general population. Although normal values vary with age, physiologic disturbances are minor until hemoglobin levels fall below 7 or 8. When the onset of anemia is gradual, subtle symptoms may be noted: pallor, weakness, tachycardia, dyspnea on exertion. As the anemia continues, or if it worsens in severity, blood flow deviates to the vital organs and tissues, with a concommittant left shift in the oxyhemoglobin dissociation curve. Ultimately, cardiac dilation and congestive heart failure may ensue.

Anemias can be differentiated efficiently by following the results of the sequence of tests depicted in bold capital letters below:

RBC MORPHOLOGY AND INDEXES
Microcytic-hypochromic anemia
   FREE ERYTHROCYTE PROTOPORPHYRIN
  Low free erythrocyte protoporphyrin (FEP)
    Thalassemia

  High free etytrhocyte protoporphyrin (FEP)
   SERUM FERRITIN
   High/normal ferritin
    Lead poisoning
    Chronic disease
    Pyridoxine deficiency
    Sideroblastic anemia
  Low ferritin
    Iron deficiency

Macrocytic-normochromic
   Megaloblastic anemia (folate, B_{12} deficiency)
   Aplastic/hypoplastic anemia
   Fanconi's anemia
   Hypothyriodism
   Congenital dyserythropoietic anemia
   Hepatic disease

Normocytic-normochromic anemia
(continued on next page)

Normocytic-nornochromic anemia
RETICULOCYTE COUNT
Low reticulocyte count
PLATELET COUNT
Low platelet count
BONE MARROW EXAMINATION
Bone marrow: Blasts present
Leukemia
Metastatic tumor
Bone marrow: Blasts absent
Aplastic/hypoplastic anemia
Lipid storage disease
High/normal platelet count
Renal disease
Infection
Inflammation
Chronic disease
Hypothryoidism
Blackfan-Diamond anemia
Transient erythroblastopenia
Congenital dyserythropoietic anemia
Protein malnutrition
High reticulocyte count
INDIRECT BILIRUBIN
Normal indirect bilirubin
blood loss
Elevated indirect bilirubin
COOMBS TEST
Positive Coombs test
Autoimmune hemolytic anemia
Isoimmune hemolytic anemia (Rh, ABO)
Incompatible transfusion
Negative Coombs test
FRAGMENTED CELLS ON PERIPHREAL SMEAR
Burr, helmet cells/schistocytes present
Hemolytic Uremic syndrome
DIC
Burr, helmet cells/schistocytes absent
OSMOTIC FRAGILITY TEST
RBC fragility test abnormal
Spherocytosis
Stomatocytosis
Elliptocytosis
Vitamin E deficiency
RBC fragility normal
HEMOGLOBIN ELECTROPHORESIS
Hb electrophoresis abnormal
Sickle cell disease
Hg SC disease
Hg5-beta-thalassemia
Hb electrophoresis normal
G-6-PD deficiency
Pyruvate kinase deficiency
Elliptocytosis
Stomatocytosis

Disease Profiles

Inadequate Production of Red Blood Cells or Hemoglobin due to:
    A. decreased red cell precusors
        1. Pure red all aplasia

Alternate Terminology
    Diamond-Blackfan Syndrome
    Congenital pure red cell anemia
    Congenital hypoplastic anemia

Etiology
    Instances of familial occurrence have been reported and males and females are affected equally, but no genetic basis currently established. Low numbers of eryrocyte colony forming units.

Pathophysiologic Abnormality
    Profound anemia by 2-6 months of age

Predisposing Conditions
    Congenital aunomalies, include triphalangeal thumbs
    Turner Syndrome phenotype with normal karyotype

Physical Findings
    Pallor
    Hepatosplemegaly
    Congestive heart failure

Laboratory Findings
    Macrocytic, normochronic anemia
    Increased Hgb F level
    Occasionally neutropenia, thrombocytopenia
    High serum erythropoetin
    Decreased reticulocyte count
    Bone marrow - markedly reduced red cell precisors
    Myeloid - erythroid ratios 10-200:1
    Elevated serum iron
    Decreased total serum iron binding capacity

Differential Diagnosis
    Convalescent phase of hemolytic anemia of the newborn
    Aplastic crisis of parovirus-like infections
    Transient erythroblastopenia

Potential Complications
    Hemosiderosis secondary to repeated transfusions
    Hepatosplenomegaly
    Leukopenia and thrombocytopenia secondary to hypersplenism
    Growth retardation
    Delayed puberty
    Diabetes mellitus secondary to hemosiderosis
    Chronic congestive heart failure
    Spontaneous remission occasionally occurs
    If no response to therapy, death occurs by the second decade

Therapeutic Plan
    Corticosteroid therapy (may be beneficial if begun early) 85-90% responsive cases may outgrow dependence on steroid therapy
    Blood transfusions to correct anemia at 4 to 8 week intervals
    Splenectomy if hypersplenism present

Clulation in patients with hemosiderosis
? bone marrow transplant

2. Acquired pure red cell anemias
    Etiology
        Serum antibody to erythropoeitin, erythroblasts
        Heme synthesis inhibitor
        Viral infections
        Exposure to chloramphenical
        Thymoma

    Predisposing Conditions
        Autoimmune disease
        Biochemical or membrane red cell defect
        Thymoma

    Laboratory Findings - Marked reduction in circulating reticulocytes elevation of serum iron

    Bone Marrow - Markedly reduced numbers of erythroid precursors

    Diagnostic Plan
        Resection of thymoma, if present
        Corticosteroids
        Immunosuppressive therapy with cyclophosphanide or azathioprine

3. Transient erythroblastopenia of childhood - severe aregenerative anemia

    Etiology
        Serum inhibitor of erythroid stem cells
        Abnormalities of erythroid stem cells
        (number of responsiveness to erythropoetin)
        Autoimmune disease directed at primitive red cell precursors

    Pathophysiology
        Slow development of anemia with reticulocytopenia in previously normal children 6
        months - 5 years of age

        Decreased numbers of red cell precursors in bone marrow

        Profile of red cell enqymes consistent with an "old" red cell population

    Laboratory Findings
        Serum iron increased
        Iron saturation increased
        Hgb F level normal
        Red cell adenosine deaminose activity normal

    Therapeutic Plan
        Spontaneous remission occurs
        Transfusions may be necessary until recovery

B. Inadequate production Despite normal numbers of red cell precursors

    4. Anemia of Chronic Disease - associated with chronic system diseases associated with infection,
    inflammation, or tissue breakdown

        Etiology
            Bronchiectasis
            Osteomyelitis
            Tuberculosis

Rheumatic fever
Rheumatoid arthritis
Ulcerative colitis
Advanced renal disease
Malignancy

Pathophysiology
Moderate decrease of red cell life span
Increased red cell destruction by hyperactive reticuloendothelial system
Relative failure of bone marrow response
Inadequate erythropoetin production
Abnormalities of iron metabolism

Symptoms
Few actual symptoms of anemia; significant signs and symptoms those of underlying disease

Laboratory Findings
Hemoglobin concentration range 6 to 9 g/dl
Usually normochronic, normocytic anemia, although wild hypochronic & microcytosis may be seen
Reticulocyte count normal or low
Leukocytosis common
Free erythrocyte protoporplyrin levels moderately elevated
Serum iron low
Normal total iron binding capacity
Serum ferritin frequently elevated
Bone marrow - normal cellularity

Therapeutic Plan
Treatment of underlying disease process

5. Physiologic Anemia of Infancy

Etiology
Infant born with higher hemoglobin and hematocrit levels than older children and adults
Progressive decline for 6-8 weeks with physiologic nadir of ~9 for full term infants

Pathophysiology
Abrupt cessation of erythropoiesis with onset of respiration
Shortened fetal red cell survival
Rapid weight gain   sizable blood volume expansion
At 2-3 months of age, when the Hgb level has dropped to 9 to 11, erythropoiesis resumes
Physiologic adaption to extrauterine life

Predisposing Conditions
Premature infant has a more exaggerated nadir, with a more rapid decline to levels of 7 to 9 by 3 to 6 weeks of age.

Therapeutic Plan
Ensure that dirt contains essential nutrients for normal heutopoeisis - esp. folic acid and vitamin E
Infrequently, transfusion may be required

C. Deficiencies of biochemical factors: macrocytic morphology

In patients with megaloblastic anemia, all rapidly proliferating cells in the body are enlarged. The postulated primary cellular abnormality is a diminished capacity to synthesize DNA. However, RNA synthesis is less affected, allowing cytoplasmic maturation and growth to continue, which accounts for cellular enlargement, neutrophils and megalcoryocytes are also enlarged, with nuclear segmentation. Megalcaryocytes may be fragmented.

Pathophysiology

Inadequate intake or absorption - polygutanis of folic acid or present in wide variety of foods and is also formed by intestinal bacteria. Conjugase enzymes in bile and the intestine lydrolize the polyglutantes prior to jejunal absorption. Folate is rapidly removed from plasma to cells and tissues for utilization, but the chief storage site is the liver. Anemia appears 3 to 6 months after initiation of deficiency.

Predisposing Conditions
　　Pregnancy
　　Hemolytic anemia
　　Congenital defect of folic acid absorption
　　Drug therapy (pheztoin, primidone, phenobarbital, methotrencili, amnepterin, pyrimethanine, trimethoprim sulfa)
　　Congenital dihydrofolate deficiency
　　Rapid growth
　　Infection
　　Ascorbic acid defiency

Symptoms
　　Irritability
　　Chronic diarrhea
　　Failure to thrive

Laboratory Findings
　　Macrocyne anemia
　　Low reticulocyte count
　　Peripheral nucleated red blood cells
　　Neutropenia
　　Hypersegmented neutrophils
　　Thrombocytopenia
　　Decreased serum folic acid (< 3ng/ml)
　　Decreased red cell folate level (< 150ng/ml)
　　Elevated LDH
　　Hypercellular bone marrow
　　Hypersegmented megalcaryocytes

Diagnostic Plan
　　therapeutic trial of folic acid replacant will differentiate it from Vitamin B_{12} deficiency.

Therapeutic Plan
　　Parenteral folic acid (50-200ng/day) will produce an adequate reticticulocyte response
　　Folic acid therapy should be continued for 3 to 4 weeks
　　Blood transfusion should be considered only in severe cases

6. Vitamin B_{12} deficiency

Vitamin B_{12} is found in virtually all animal tissues, and is related by protein digestion. gastric intrinsic factor then binds it, and the B_{12}-intrinsic factor complex adheres to epithelial receptor sites of the ileum, where it is subsequently absorbed.

Alternate Terminology
　　Pernicious anemia

Etiology
　　Inadequate intake (rare)
　　Failure of gastric secretion of intrinic factor
　　B_{12} - intrinic factor inhibition or consumption
　　Ileal receptor site dysfunction

Predisposing Conditions
　　Congenital inability to secrete
　　Transcobalamin dificiency (gastric intrinsic factor autosomal recessive)
　　Malabsorption (with or without gastric mucosal atrophy and achlorlycluria)
　　Familial syndrome of cutaneous candidosis, hypo parathroidism & other endocrine deficiences (make antibodies to intrinsic factor and parietal cells)

Ismerlund Syndrome
Regional enteritis
Gastrointestinal tuberculosis
Diphyllobothrium latum infestation of small intestine
Diverticular disease
Duplications of small intestine

Physical Findings
Anemia
Irritability
Anorexia
Listlessness
Smooth, red, painful tongue
Ataxia, paresthesias, hyporeflexia, babinski response, clonus, coma

Laboratory Findings
Macrocytic anemia
Hypersegmented neutrophils
Serum B_{12} levels less than 100pg/ml
Serum LDH increased
Serum iron normal or elevated
Moderate elevation of serum bilirubin
Increased methylmalonic acid secretion in urine

Schilling Test - ingestion of B_{12} bound to a radioisotope. In the normal individual, the radioactive vitamin is absorbed and none is excreted in the urine. A large dose of nonradioactive B_{12} is then injected parenterally and subsequently 10 to 30% of the radioactive vitamin will be present in the urine. Patients with peruicious anemia will excrete less than 2% (absence of intrinsic factor) when the test is performed. If deficiency is suspected to be due to gastrointestinal disease or malfunctioning receptor sites, intrinsic factor can be given with a second oral dose of radioactive B_{12} , and no improvement in absorption will be seen.

Treatment
With neurologic involvement, 1mg of vitamin B_{12} should be administered daily for at least 2 weeks.
Maintenance therapy with 1mg of vitamin B_{12} should be administered intramuscularly on a monthly basis. Oral therapy is contraindicated.
With trausobalamin defienciency, massive parenteral doses of vitamin B_{12} are required.

7. Orotic Aciduria - Deficiency of ortotactic phosphoriozl transferase and orotidine - 5 - phosphate

A defect in pyrimdine synthesis which decarboxylase is associated with severe megaloblastic anemia, neutropenia and excretion of orotic acid crystals in the urine.

Physical and mental retardation are frequently associated.
The anemia does not respond to vitamin B_{12} or folatic administration, but may be treated with the urologic acid precursor, uridine or yeast

Autosomal recessive.

Microcytic morphology
A. Iron deficiency anemia

Most common anemia of infants and children, whose diets frequently contain food low in iron. Dietary sources are necessary for the prevention of iron deficiency anemia, and in infants on non-iron fortified formula, it can develop very rapidly.

Pathophysiology
The average newborn infant has iron stores approximately one tenth that of an adult, the majority of which is present as circulating hemoglobin. Neonatal hemoglobin falls rapidly in the first 3 to 4 months of life and the iron reclaimed from this process is available for red cell production for 6 to 9 months. After that time, it

is fairly common, primarily in infants who consume large amounts of non-iron supplented milk and carbohydrates.

Blood loss must be ruled out as another cause
1. Peptic ulcer
2. Meckel's diverticulum
3. Intestinal polyp
4. Intestinal hemangionia
5. Chronic intestinal blood loss secondary to cow's milk protein

Clinical manifestations
pallor
irritability
anorexic
systolic murmur common
splenomegaly (10-15%)
Pica
decreased attention span, alertness and ability to learn

Laboratory Findings
Low serum ferritin
Increased total iron binding capacity
Decreased percent saturation of iron
Increased free erythrocyte protoporphyrins
Microcytic hypochromic morphology on peripheral smear as disease progresses
Reticulocyte count normal or minimally elevated
Thrombocytosis or thrombocytopenic
Hypercellular bone marrow with erythroid hyperplasia

Differential Diagnosis
Lead poisoning
Beta thalasseuria trait
Alpha thalasseuria trait
Anemia of chronic disease

Therapy
Oral administration of ferrous iron salts (6mg/lg of elemental iron in 3 divided doses) between meds
Limitation of milk consumption
blood transfusion for severe anemia only

B. Sideroblastic anemias

Multiple entities caused by defects of iron or neuroglobin metabolism (Insert A)
Congenital - x-linked recessive
Acquired - alcoholism, multiple inflammatory and malignant diseases

Laboratory Findings
Increased serum iron
Ringed sideroblasts (nucleated)
red blood cells with a perinuclear halo of hemosiderin)
microcytic anemia

Treatment
May respond partially to pyridoxine

C. Lead poisoning

Alternate terminology
plumbism

Pathophysiology
Ingestion of lead from air, food, beverages, household dust and paints can cause toxic effects in the CNS, peripheral venous system, bone marrow erythroid cells and kidney

Partial inhibition of hemoglobin synthesis occurs causing a microcytic
hypochromic anemia

Clinical Manifestations
Hyperirritability
Anorexia
Decreased activity
Intermittent vomiting and abdominal pain
Constipation
Encephalopathy
Ataxia
Seizures

Laboratory Findings
High blood lead level
high free erythrocyte protophoryrin level
microcytic anemia
basophilic stippling of bone marrow normoblasts
erythroid hyperplasia
reticulocytosis

Differential Diagnosis
Other microcytic anemia
Seizure disorder
Mental retardation
Behavioral disorders
Cerebral and abdominal crisis of sickle cell disease

Treatment
Separation of child from sources of lead
Deleading of environment
Chelation therapy with Ca EDTA, (edathamil calcium disodium)
DMSA (meso-2, 3-dimercaptosuccine acid)

In cases of acute encephalopathy, BAL + CaEDTA is recommended

HEMOLYTIC ANEMIAS

Hemolytic anemia results from shortened total red blood cell survival, either due to an abnormality in the red cell itself or secondary to extrinsic factors which cause red blood cell destruction. The bone marrow responds to the anemia with increased activity and a marked reticulocytosis. Marrow hyperplasia may expand medullary bone, causing characteristic radiographic findings. Indirect hyperbilirubinemia without jaundice, as well as bilirubin gallstone formation early in life may be noted. Children with hemolytic anemias may develop bone marrow failure and aplastic crisis during parvovirus infection, causing a profound life-threatening anemia.

A. Intrinsic Causes - membrane defects
1. Hereditary splenocytosis

Congenital hemolytic anemia
Congenital acholuric jaundice

This disease is usually transmitted as an autosomal dominant, although occasional cases have an autosomal recessive hereditary pattern. 25% of cases occur as a spontaneous irritation. Spectrin, a protein which the stabilizing factor for the red cell membrane, is defective or decreased in this disease state. Affected red cells show increased sodium absorption which increases intra-cellular volume, distorting the red cell shape. The spleen removes the defective red cells, causing the anemia.

Clinical Manifestations
Anemia in the newborn
Hyperbilirubinemia in the newborn
Moderate expansion of medullary bone in the skull
Splenomegaly
Mild jaundice
Bilirubin gallstones

Aplastic crisis with parvovirus infection

Laboratory Findings
Anemia
Hyperbilirubinemia
Reticulocytosis
Typical spherocyte on peripheral smear
Elevated MCHC
Bone marrow erythroid hyperplasia
Osmotic fragility

Differential Diagnosis
Acquired spherocytosis (other hemolytic states)
ABO incompatibility (in the newborn)
Elliptocytosis

Treatment
Splenectomy is curative, but should be deferred until the child is 5 to 6 years old if possible.

2. Hereditary elliptocytosis

May have elliptocytosis with or without hemolysis.

There is a genetic basis, but it is not yet well-defined, although one gene is sometimes found linked to the Rh locus.

Variant - hereditary pyropailcilocytosis - red cells unstable in heat (Children seem to have inherited an elliptocytic gene from one parent and a different, abnormal gene from another parent)

On peripheral smear, they have elliptocytes, spherocytes, red blood cell fragments and marked microcytosis.

Clinical Manifestations
Neonatal jaundice on occasion
Anemia
Jaundice
Splenomegaly
Radiographic osseus changes
Cholelithiasis in later childhood
Occasional aplastic crisis

Laboratory Findings
Elliptocytes, bizarre poikilocytes, microcytes, spherocytes or peripheral smear
Increased reticulocyte count
Erythroid hyperplasia

Treatment
Splenectomy helpful but not curative.

3. Paroxysmal Nocturnal Hemoglobinuria (PNP)

PND is a usual chronic anemia caused by an acquired dysplastic defect of the red cell membrane that makes it susceptible to complement mediated hemolysis. The hemolysis is intravascular rather than in the spleen and is frequently exacerbated by sleep. Chronic thrombocytopenia and/or leukopenia may be present, as well as occasional hypoplasia of the bone marrow or aplastic parcypopenia. Iron may be lost in the urine.

Clinical Manifestations
Anemia
Susceptibility to pyogenic infections, and thromboembolisms
Abdominal and back pain
Headache

Laboratory Findings
Positive Ham test
Positive sucrose lysis test
Markedly reduced levels of red blood cell acetyclolinesterase
Reduced levels of "decay accelerating factor" diagnostic

Treatment
Splenectomy does not alter the disease process
Bone marrow transplant has been useful.
Prolonged anticoagulation therapy if thromboembolic events occur
Iron replacement may be necessary

4. Hereditary/Acquired Stomatocytosis

This is an unusual condition caused by extreme membrane permeability to cations which may be associated with hemolytic anemia. red blood cells are swollen and cup-shaped, and show a slit in the center of the red blood cell in place of central pallor, acquired stomatocytosis may be seen with liver disease and other disorders.

Therapy
Splenectomy may be of some benefit in severe cases.

B. Intrinsic Cause - red cell Enzymatic defects
1. Pyruvate kinase deficiency

Autosomal recessive condition which demonstrates either a significant reduction in red blood cell pyruvate kinase or an abnormal enzyme with decreased activity. Decreased ATP causes a reduction in intracellular potassium leading to a shortened red cell life span.

Clinical Manifestations
Some children may develop a severe congenital hemolytic anemia, whereas other may have only a mild anemia frequently diagnosed later in life.
Jaundice with kernicterus on occasion
Pallor
Splenomegaly

Laboratory Findings
Elevated reticulocyte count
Peripheral smear - macrocytosis, pylenocytosis, polychromatophilia
Marked reduction of red blood cell
Pyruvate kinase activity - diagnostic
Heterozygous carriers demonstrated moderately reduced levels of pyruvate kinase activity

Treatment
Exchange transfusion may be necessary with significant neonatal hyperbilirubinemia
Transfusion
Splenectomy by 5 to 6 years of age if anemic is severe (not curative, but reduce severity of disease)

2. Glucose - 6 - phosphate dehydroglucose Deficiency (G-G-PD)

This disease is caused by abnormal synthesis of G-G-PD, which over 100 different enzyme variants have been found at this time. Because of this, the severity of the disease process is variable. Because red blood cell GGPD synthesis is mediated by genes located on the X chromosome, it occurs more frequently in males than females. People of Mediterranean, African and Asian descent are at increased risk for this enzymatic defect.

Ingestion of antioxidant drugs (drtipyretics, sulfonamides, antimalarials and napthaquinolones) as well as fava beans (a Mediterranean staple) cause a hemolytic anemia whose severity is influenced by the amount of the substance ingested, the agent and the patient's enzyme deficiency.

Clinical Manifestations
Neonatal jaundice and kevuicterus may occur, but the most dramatic anemia develops with exposure to one of the above mentioned agents.

48 to 96 hours after ingestion of an inciting agent, the patient develops hemolysis. In severe cases, the hemoglobin concentration may decrease by as much as 70%. Hemoglobimia and jaundice may be present, and death may ensue if hemolysis is severe and supportive therapy is not available.

Pregnant women who ingest one of these agents may cause hemolytic anemia and jaundice in an affected infant.

Premature black infants may develop spontaneous hemolysis.

Laboratory Findings

Anemia
Unstained peripheral smears may show Heiz bodies in the red blood cells in the early illness
Variants may be noted by hemoglobin electrophoresis
Reduced G-G PD red blood cell activity (10% of normal or less)
Reticulocytosis in the recovery phase.

Treatment
Avoidance of agents which cause hemolysis
Supportive therapy, including transfusion
Spontaneous recovery occurs if the patient survives.

C. Intrinsic Cause - structural abnormalities of hemoglobin

1 Sickle cell disease
Over 500 hemoglobin variants have been identified, the majority of which do not cause clinically significant disease, Sickle hemoglobin, or hemoglobin S occurs when the B chain has valine substitution for glutaminic acid in the sixth position. As long as the hemoglobin is well-oxygenated, it functions normally. When it is exposed to lower than normal partial pressures of oxygen, a polymerization defect occurs which causes rigidity of the hemoglobin. red blood cells containing affected hemoglobin S are brittle and poorly deformable, leading to premature destruction and clumping of the cells which can cause vascular occlusion. Heterozygotes for this disorder are minimally affected and show increased resistion to invasion of malarial parasites (sickle trait). Homozygotes have sickle cell anemia, which has protein manifestations.

Clinical Manifestations
Affected newborns are usually asymptomatic, because of the presence of hemoglobin F. By approximately 4 months of age, most hemoglobin F has been replaced by hemoglobin S and anemia results. There are three clinical entities which comprise acute exacerbations of the disease.

Hand-foot syndrome or acute dactylitis is commonly the first presentation, occurring in infants and small children. These children have painful, frequently symmetric swelling of the hands and feet, caused by ischemic necrosis of the small bones due to the rapidly expanding bone marrow.

Vaso-occlusive crisis
Most common type of crisis
May be precipitated by infection or develop spontaneously
Caused by distal ischemia and tissue infarction
Older children may have large joint manifestations, or abdominal pain secondary to infarction of abdominal structures. Cerebral and pulmonary infarctions may occur as well.

Sequestration Crisis
Large volumes of blood pool in the liver and spleen with subsequent circulatory collapse. The etiology is unknown. With supportive care, the sequestered blood may be remobilized. The severity of the episodes are related to the degree of splenic autoinfarction.

Aplastic Crisis
Can occur when there is supression of the marrow by viral infestions.

A. Eugene Osburn

Developmental Considerations

Bilious vomiting should not be attributed to gastroenteritis in the child. Its presence should prompt a search for obstructive lesions in this age group.

Gastroesophageal Reflux
A common problem to some degree in the first year of life.
Sandifer syndrome is GER associated with torticollis and back arching.
24 hour esophageal pH monitoring is the most definitive diagnostic test.
May be a cause of neonatal apnea.
Medical treatment is:
>> Elevating head after feeding (in infant seat)
>> Bethanechol to increase esophageal peristalsis, gastric emptying, and lower esophageal tone
>> metoclopramide to increase gastric empting and increase lower esophageal tone
>> H$_2$ blockers and antiacids

Surgical treatment:
>> Nissen fundoplication

Pyloric Stenosis
More common in males
Nonbilous vomiting begins 2 to 4 weeks of life, which becomes projectile in nature.
When significant, it is associated with weight loss, hypokalemic metabolic alkalosis, paradoxic aciduria and dehyration. Hyperbilirubinemia is also common.
Must be differentiated from Congenital Adrenal Hyperplasia (CAD) which can present at same age. CAD has hyperkalemia, and a metabolic acidosis.
Diagnosis is made by palpation of a gastric olive-shaped mass, ultrasound identification of the hypertrophied muscle or by a string sign on barrium upper GI.
Treatment is pyloromyotomy after fluid and electrolyte derrangements are corrected.

Congenital Malformations

Cleft lip/palate
Caused by multiple genetic as well as environmental factors.
Recurrence risk in siblings is 3-4%
Children with cleft palate are at increased risk for recurrent otitis media.

Pierre Robin syndrome
High arched or cleft palate, micrognathia and glossoptosis.
Airway obstruction and feeding problems may occur until the mandible grows enough for the problem to resolve.

Tracheoesophageal fistulaes
Esophageal atresia with communication via a fistula with the trachea occurs in all but the H-type in which there is a communication without esophageal atresia. The other types are classified according to which part of the atretic esophagus communicates with the esophagus.
Forty percent have associated anomalies; cardiac anomalies are the most common.
Early clues to this disorder are polyhydramnois and excessive drooling at birth.

Cough, choking and cyanosis with feeding is characteristic of symptomatic types.

Ophalocele

High incidence of other associated malformations.

Beckwith-Wiedemann syndrome (exophthalmos, macroglossia, gigantism, hypoglycemia; increased incidence of Wilm's tumors later in life in this syndrome)

Umbilical hernia

More common in premature and black infants.

Increased incidence in hypothyroidism.

Facial defects less than 0.5 cm usually spontaneously close by age 2 years; defects 0.5-1.5 cm spontaneously close by age 4 years.

Abdominal binders (coins, etc. taped over defect) does not increase healing rate.

Duodenal obstruction

May be due to atresia (complete obstruction) or stenosis (partial obatruction due to a web, band, or annular pancreas) in the neonate.

More common in premature and infants with Down's syndrome.

Characteristic "double bubble" on abdominal X-ray due to gastric and duodenal gaseous distention.

With complete obstruction, polyhydramnois may be present and bilous vomitus begins within a few hours after feeding.

Jejunal/Ileal obstruction

Meconuim ileus with or without atresia is associated with cystic fibrosis.

Polyhyramnois is present in complete atresia.

Bile stained vomitus within 24-48 hours after feeding.

X-ray of the abdomen shows dilated loops of small bowel, with absence of air in the colon.

Malrotation/Volvulus

The majority of infants with this anomaly present with symptoms within the first month of life.

Bilous vomiting and abdominal distention suggests obstruction.

Bloody stools may occur is volvulus results in bowel ischemia.

Meckel Diverticulum

The most common anomaly of the gastrointestinal tract.

It is due to the the presence of a vestigial remnant of the omphalomesenteric duct.

Gastric tissue is common in symptomatic cases because it causes acid secretion and ulceration.

Presenting clinical manifestations include: painless rectal bleeding, intestinal obstruction (due to intussusception or volvulus) or diverticulitis (mimics appendicitis).

Hirschsprung Disease (Congenital Aganglionic Megacolon)

An aganglionic segment of variable length of the colon may be present.

Three times more common in males.

Most are limited to the rectosigmoid colon.

Diagnosis should be suspected in the infant who fails to pass meconium in the first 24 hours, or who requires repeated rectal stimulation to pass stools.

The diagnosis may escape detection until later in childhood, at which time, abdominal distention, failure to thrive, anemia, palpable stool in the abdomen with an empty rectal vault may be clues.

The patients usually have a history of small ribbon like stools. Children with functional megacolon have encopresis, large infrequent stools.

Diagnosis is suggested by an unpreped barium enema; it is confirmed by rectal biopsy.

Toxic megacolon is a serious potential complication and is heralded by fever, abdominal distention, pain and diarrhea.

Pathophysiologic Manifestations

```
┌─────────────────────────────────────────────────────────────────┐
│                                                                   │
│              Common Causes of Abdominal Pain by Age               │
│                                                                   │
```

Infant	Child	Adolescent
Necrotizing entercolitis	Gastroenteritis	Pelvic inflammatory disease
Volvulus	Appendicitis	Ectopic Pregnancy
Incarcerated hernia	Henoch-Schonlein purpura	Inflammatory bowel disease
Hirschsprung's disease	Urinary tract infection	Testicular torsion
Intussusception	Hemolytic-Uremic Syndrome	Biliary disease
Infantile colic	Constipation	
Perforation (R/O abuse)	Ulcers	
	Pancreatitis	
	Functional pain	

Pathophysiologic Mechanisms of Diarrhea

Mechanism	pathophysiology	Stool characteristics
Secretory	decreased absorption; increased secretion	Watery; Normal osmolality: osmols= 2 X (Na$^+$ + K$^+$)
Osmotic	Maldigestion; transport defects	Watery; Acidic: + reducing substances; Increased osmolality: osmols > 2 X (Na$^+$ + K$^+$)
Increased peristalsis	Decreased Transient time	Fecal-like; Stimulated by gastrocolic reflex
Decreased mucosal area	Decreased functional capacity	Watery
Mucosal invasion	Inlfammation; decreased colonic readsoption; increased motility	Blood and increased WBC

Common Causes of Acute Diarrhea by age group

Infancy
Gastroenteritis
Overfeeding
Systemic infection
Antibiotic-associated

Childhood
Gastroenteritis
Food poisoning
Systemic infection
Antibiotic-associated

Adolescence
Gastroenteritis
Food poisoning
Antibiotic associated

Common Causes of Chronic Diarrhea by age group

Infancy
Postinfectious
Secondary disaccharidase
  deficiency
Milk protein intolerance
Irritable colon syndrome
Cystic fibrosis
Celiac disease
Short bowel syndrome

Childhood
Postinfectious
Secondary disaccharidase
  deficiency
Irritable bowel syndrome
Celiac disease
Lactose intolerance
Giardiasis

Adolescence
Inflammatory bowel
  disease
Lactose intolerance
Giardiasis
Laxative abuse

Causes of Gastrointestnal Maladsorption

Defective digestion
    Pancreatic deficiency
        cystic fibrosis
        pancreatitis
        Schwachmann syndrome
    Bile salt deficiency
        Biliary atresia
        Cholestasis
        Hepatitis
        Cirrhosis
        Bacterial decongugation

Defective absorption
    Primary absorption defects
        Glucose-galactose malabsorption
        abetalipoproteinemia
        cystinuria
        Hartnup disease
    Decreased mucosal surface area
        Crohn disease
        malnutrition
        short bowel syndrome
    Small intestinal disease
        Celiac disease
        tropical sprue
        girariasis
        lymphoma
        Allergic enteritis

Infestations
        Hookworm
        Tapeworm
        Opportunistic infections in AIDS

Lymphatic obstruction
        Lymphangiectasia
        Whipple disease
        lymphoma

Causes of Upper Gastrointestinal Bleeding by Age Group

Neonate
Swallowed
maternal blood
Gastritis
Esophagitis
Congenital blood
dyscrasia
Vascular
malformation

Infant
Gastritis
Esophagitis
Stress ulcer
Mallory-Weiss
tear
Duplication
Vascular
malformation

Child
Esophageal varices
Peptic ulcer disease
Stress ulcer
Gastritis
Mallory-Weiss tear
Foreign body
Esophagitis

Adolescent
Esophageal
varices
Peptic ulcer
Gastritis
Mallory-Weiss
tear
Esophagitis
Stress ulcer

Causes of Lower Gastrointestinal Bleeding by Age Group

Neonate
Anal fissure
Upper GI bleeding
Volvulus
Necrotizing
enterocolitis
Swallowed maternal
blood
Infectious colitis
Milk allergy
Blood dyscrasia
Duplication

Infant
Anal fissure
Intussusception
Meckel's
diverticulum
Infectious diarrhea
Milk allergy
Duplication
Pseudomembranous
colitis

Child
Polyps
Anal fissure
Meckel's
diverticulum
Infectious diarrhea
Henoch-Schonlein
Purpura
Hemolytic-Uremic
Syndrome
Intussusception
Pseudomembranous
colitis

Adolescent
Polyps
Hemorrhoids
Inflammatory
bowel disease
Infectious
diarrhea

A. Eugene Osburn

Developmental Considerations

Nephrogenesis is not complete until 36 weeks gestation. Therefore, premature infants have compromised renal functional capacity compaired to term infants.

Fetal urine is excreted into the amniotic fluid. Olgiohydraminos will result from inadequate urine output from a fetus.

Inadequate aminotic fluid is associated with pulmonary hypoplasia which may be incompatible with life.

Potter's syndrome, which is characterized by a typical facial appearance, low set ears and pulmonary hypoplasia can be a result of severe intrauterine oliguria or anuria.

Intrauterine urinary tract obstruction can cause renal dysplasia with resulting renal insufficiency from which the infant may not completely recover.

Serum Creatinine for the first 5 days of life in the newborn reflects the mother's creatinine level, not the infant's renal function.

Glomerular filtration rate: The GFR at birth is 20 to 30 ml/1.73 m^2/min.
The GFR doubles (40 to 60) by 2 weeks after birth.
The GFR should reach adult levels (120 ml/1.73m^2/min.) by age 2 years.

Clearance of drugs cleared by renal excretion may cause toxicity if given to infants in doses based on expected adult level GFR.

Urine concentrating and diluting ability: Newborn kidneys can only concentrate urine to 1/2 that of adults. i.e. 600-700 mosm/kg, instead of 1200-1400 mosm/kg. Newborns can dilute urine to adult levels (50 mosm/kg), but total water load excretion is limited by decreased GFR's.

Electrolyte regulation: Newborns can neither conserve nor effectively excrete excess sodium. As a result, potassium and hydrogen secretion are impaired.

Diagnostic Modalities

Urinalysis
    Specific Gravity
        1.002 relectes a maximally dilute urine and correlates with a urine osmolality
        of 50 mosm/kg. 1.035 (1200 mosm/kg osmolality) reflects maximally
        concentrated urine. Isotherunia, or a specific gravity of 10.10 (osmolality of
        300 mosm/kg), reflects neither concentration nor dilution of filtered serum .
    Urine dipsticks
        Commonly available dipsticks measure albumin, glucose, ketones bilirubin,
        blood, and leukocyte esterase. Positive blood in the absence of RBC's in the
        microscopic occurs from free hemaglobin and myoglobin in the urine.
    Urine microscopy
        Useful for identifying RBC;s WBC;s, casts crystals and bacteria. The presence
        of epithelial cells should also be noted since large numbers may reflect a non-
        clean catch specimen. The urine must be examined as soon as possible after
        voiding to accurately identify microscopic components since cells and casts
        can lyse in urine.
    Urine electrolytes
        Sodium
            Maximal conservation is reflected by a value of < 20 mEq/L.
            In renal failure the urine sodium is > 50 mEq/L.
        Chloride
            Maximum conservation is reflected by a value < 10 mEq/L.
            The significance of urine chloride concentrations must be intrepeted
            in light of the patient's acid-base status.
        Potassium
            Maximal tubular conservation is reflected in a value of < 20 mEq/L.
            Low values may reflect a total body deficit of potassium, regardless of
            the serum potassium level, although the urine potassium also reflects
            renin activity and tubular response to that activity. Increased renin
            activity, (whether physiologically or pathologically elevated) will
            increase potassium excretion. Renin can be elevated in response to
            hyvolemic states even in presence of total body or serum potassium
            deficits.

Glomerular function tests
    Blood urea nitrogen (BUN)
        Dependent on dietary protein intake.
        Begins to rise when GFR < 50% normal.
        Elevation also caused by blood in GI tract.
        Upon restoration of normal renal function, elevated BUN levels should
        decrease by 1/2 it's level every 16 hours.
    Serum creatinine (Cr)
        Not influenced by protein intake. The nomal value can be estimated by the
            formula: $Cr = 0.004 \times$ height in centimeters.
    BUN/Cr ratio
        Normal: 15:1 (range 10:1 to 20:1)
        Prerenal azotemia: > 40:1
    Glomerular filtration rate (GFR)
        The most common method used for measuring the GFR is by calculating the
            Creatinine Clearence (C_{Cr}).

Creatinine Clearance (C_{Cr}) calculation:

$$C_{Cr} = \frac{\text{Urine Cr x Urine Volume}}{\text{Plasma Cr}}$$

$$\text{Corrected } C_{Cr} = \frac{\text{Patient's } C_{Cr} \text{ x } 1.73 \text{ m}^2}{\text{Patient's surface area}}$$

$$\text{Simplified } C_{Cr} = \frac{\text{K x Height in cm}}{\text{Plasma Cr in mg/dl}}$$

K = 0.45 under 1 year age
K = 0.55 over 1 year age

Renal tubular function tests

Tubular function tests can help differientate between causes of olguria due to decreased GFR in the presence of tubules with normal functional capability (prerenal azotemia) and those accompied by more diffuse renal damage (renal failure azotemia). In prerenal azotemia the FEN_a is low (< 1%), whereas, in renal failure azotemia, it is high (> 7%).

Fractional excretion of sodium (FENa) calculation:

$$FENa = \frac{\text{urine Na x serum Cr}}{\text{urine Cr x serum Na}} \text{ x } 100\%$$

Imaging tests

Ultrasound

Non-invasive. It can identify the size, shape, and density of the kidneys, but is not helpful for assessing renal function.

Intravenous pyleography

Should rarely be used in children since the availibility of radionuclide scanning. Besides the potential of allergic reactions to the dye, it's tonicity can precipate renal failure. It does provide better delineation of caliceal structures than radionuclide scans.

Voiding cystourethrography

Useful for identifying vesicoureteral reflux. The same information can be obtained more safely with radionuclide scanning, except for visualization of the urethra.

Radionuclide scanning

Can provide as assesment of GFR in each kidney as well as assessment of tubular activity depending on which isotope is used. When instilled into the bladder instead of being given IV, it can be used for cystograms, but not visualization of the urethra.

Serum complement (C_3)

Hypocomplementemia can be found in the following conditions:

Poststreptococcal glomerulonephritis (should return to normal within 8 weeks)

Systemic lupus erythematosus (decreased complement reflects exacerbation of active lupus nephritis)

Membranoproliferative glomerulonephtitis (the complement level remains persistently low)

Chronic infections (decreased complement reflects vasculitis which can involve glomerilar interary)

Hereditary complement deficiencies (can also be associated with vasculitis)

Renal biopsy

May be necessary if a histologic diagnosis is needed. It is generally not needed in uncomplicated cases of Lipoid Nephrosis of Childhood, nor in acute glomerulonephritis.

Indications for dialysis

In acute renal failure, the level of BUN and/or Creatinine are not the determining factors in deciding when to initiate dialysis.

Dialysis is initiated in acute renal failure to control:
Acidosis
Metabolic
Electrolyte abnormalities
Especially hyperkalemia (which may not be controlled by diet alone when the GFR drops below 5 ml/min/1.73m^2)
Fluid overload
Hypertension
Congestive heart failure
Pulmonary edema
Uremic complications
Encephalopathy
Pericarditis or pericardial effusion
Coagulation disturbances

In chronic renal failure, dialysis will generally be required when the GFR falls to < 0.1-0.15 ml/min/kg (7-11 ml/min/1.73m^2)

Pathophysiologic Manifestations

Oliguria

May be a normal physiologic response to water and/or salt depletion, i.e.prerenal olgiuria, or a reflection of renal failure. The concommitant presence of azotemia reflects a process beyond the kidney's ability to compensate.

Differientiation of prerenal vs. renal oliguria

TEST	PRERENAL	RENAL
FE_{Na}	< 1%	> 3%
BUN/Cr ratio	>20:1	< 10:1
Urine Specific Gravity	> 1.015	< 1.010

Edema

Edema formation requires an excessive accumulation of both sodium and salt. The kidneys may cause edema due to ineffective excretion of sodium and water or through their enhanced readsorption either to replinish a decreased intravascular volume or in response to minerlaocoritcoid excesses.

Causes of generalized edema

Inability to excrete sodium and water load
Glomerular lesions resulting in decreased GFR
Excess salt intake
Loss of plasma oncotic pressure
Nephrotic syndrome
Protein-losing enteropathy
Chronic protein malnutrition
Decreased cardiac output
Congestive heart failure
Pericardial effusion
Excessive mineralcorticoid activity
Hyper-renin states
Hyperaldersteronism
Corticosteroid excess
Hepatic Failure

Polyuria

Water conservation is dependent on Antidiuretic Hormone (ADH) and it's effect on end organ sites on the distal renal tubules.

Causes of Polyuria:

    Central diabetes insipidus (ADH deficiency)
        Idiopathic diabetes insipidus
        Acquired diabetes insipidus
            CNS infections
            Pituitary trauma
    Nephrogenic diabetes insipidus (end organ defect)
        Hereditary form
        Acquired forms
            Intersitial nephritis
            Sickle cell disease
            Chronic renal failure
            Hypokalemia
            Papillary necrosis
    Psychogenic polydipsia
    Osmotic loads
        Glucose
            uncontrolled diabetes mellitus
            iatrogenic hyperglycemia
        Mannitol
    Volume expansion
        IV fluids
        Diuretic phase of resolving acute renal failure

Hypertension

Renal diseases are the most common ogranic cause of hypertension in children.
The finding of hypertension demands evaluation of renal funciton. Hypertension may be due to salt and water retention, excess renin or both as the result of a renal disease. In general hypertension should be further evaluated if the blood pressure is greater than 120/80 in infants, 140/90 in children or 160/100 in adolscents, or is associated with the following signs of end organ insult:

End Organ	Manifestation of hypertensive insult
CNS	Hypertensive encephalopathy, Increased intracranial pressure Headache, seizures, altered sensorium
Heart	Congestive heart failure, Pulmonary edema, Ventricular hypertrophy
Kidney	Proteinuria, decreased GFR

Hematuria
    Normal number of RBC'/HPF in urine: < 5

Proteinuria
    Normal protein excretion: < 4 mg/m^2/hour
    Nephrotic syndrome producing rate of protein excretion: > 40 mg/m^2/hour

Differientiating the cause of proteinuria and/or hematuria can be facilitated by consideration of associated findings in the patient:

Proteinuria without hematuria or edema:
Transient proteinuria
Orthostatic proteinuria
"Allergic" phenomena
Pre-nephrotic
Focal segmental glomerulosclerosis

Proteinuria with edema and no hematuria:
Mininal lesion nephrotic syndrome
Focal segmental glomerulosclerosis

Proteinuria with edema and hematuria:
Acute glomerulonephritis
Minimal lesion nephrotic syndrome
Chronic and/or progressive glomerulonephtitis
Lupus Nephritis
Membranoproliferative glomerulonephritis
Hereditary glomerulonephritis

Proteinuria with hematuria and no edema:
Acute glomerulonephritis
Idiopathic hypercalciuria
IgA Nephropathy
Reflux nephropathy
Acute interstitial nephritis
Urinary tract infection
Cystic kidneys

Hematuria without proteinuria or edema:
Beign transient hematuria
Trauma
Idiopathic hypercalciuria
Nephrolithiasis
Urethral foreign body

Enuresis

90% of children stop bedwetting by the age of 5 years. Urinary tract infections and idiopathic hypercalcinuria need to be ruled out. Arginine vasopressin (DDAVP) may be useful in some children. Tricylic antidpressants have been used, but have potentially dangerous side effects, and are not recommended.

Nephrotic Syndrome

The nephrotic syndrome is characterized by **proteinuria, hypoptoteinemia, edema, and hyperlipidemia.** If urinary protein loss exceeds 40 mg/m^2/hour for an adequate length of time, hypoprotienemia (due to the liver's inability to replinish the loss), edema (due to decreased oncotic pressure) and hyperlipidemia (a by-product of the increased liver synthesis of protein) will ensue.

Causes of Nephrotic Syndrome

Primary glomerular involvment
Without inflammatory glomerular changes
MINIMAL CHANGE NEPHROTIC SYNDROME
FOCAL SEGMENTAL GLOMERULOSCLEROSIS
CONGENITAL NEPHROTIC SYNDROME
With inflammatory glomerular changes
ACUTE POSTSTEPTOCOCCAL GLOMERULONEPHRITIS
MEMBRANOPROLIFERATIVE GLOMERULONEPHRITIS
MEMBRANOUS NEPHROPATHY
MESANGIAL PROLIFERATIVE GLOMERULONEPHTITIS

Glomerular insults secondary to systemic diseases with vasculitis
Inflammatory diseases
SYSTEMIC LUPUS ERYTHEMATOSUS
HENOCH-SCHOLEIN PURPURA
SYSTEM VASCULITIS
HEMOLYTIC-UREMIC SYNDROME
Infections
Viral infections
HEPATITIS
CYTOMEGALOVIRUS
EPSTEIN-BARR VIRUS
Bacterial infections
SHUNT NEPHRITIS
SUBACUTE BACTERIAL ENDOCARDITIS
Parasitic infections
MALARIA
Malignant diseases
LYMPHOMAS
LEUKEMIAS
SOLID TUMORS
Metabolic diseases
DIABETES MELLITUS
HYPOTHYROIDISM
Exogenous toxins and poisons
MEDICATIONS
HEAVY METALS
VENOMS
Other disorders
SICKLE CELL DISEASE
RENAL VEIN THOMBOSIS

Renal Failure

May occur with or without decreased urine output, i.e. oliguric or non-oliguric renal failure. The result is inability of the kidney to maintain water, electrolyte and acid-base homeostasis, or to eliminate waste products of metabolism.

Classification of the degree of renal failure

Acute tubular necrosis

Potentially transient renal insult, which if promptly reversed by judicious fluid supplimentation and/or low dose dopamine (5mcg/kg/min) may not progress to frank renal failure.

Acute Renal Failure

Compromise of renal function to the extent the following complications can develop:

Complication	Result
water retention	dilutional hyponatremia causing coma, seizures, lethargy
sodium retention	fluid overload causing: edema, hypertension, cardiac failure
Hyperkalemia	Cardiac rhythm and conduction disturbances
Metabolic acidosis	Impaired cellular metabolism
Uremic syndrome	accumulation of "uremic toxins" which eventually causes: anorexia, encephalopathy pericarditis, prolonged bleeding time

Dialysis may be required to support the patient until renal function has improved.

Chronic Renal Failure

In addition to the complications seen in acute renal failure, chronic renal failure is characterized by:

Malnutrition and growth failure. Dialysis can permit adequate calorie and protein intake to promote growth.

Renal osteodystrophy (Renal Rickets). Inaddition to added dietary Vitamin D and phosphate binders such as calcium carbonate, amelioration of this complication may require parathyroidectiomy.

Anemia. An effective synthetic erythropoitin is now available which avoids the necessity of blood transfusions for this complication.

Hypertension. If present, treatment will be required to prevent additional insult to the kidney as well as other organs.

Hyperkalemia. Dietary potassium restriction is generally not needed until the GFR has decreased to less than 5 ml/min/1.73m^2.

May not require dialysis until the GFR has decreased to < 7-11 ml/min/1.73m^2.

End Stage Renal Disease

Treatment will require chronic dialysis (hemodialysis or peritoneal dialysis) or renal transplant

Causes of renal failure

Prerenal

Decreased perfusion of the kidneys with resultant
impaired substrate delivery to renal cells:

Hypotension
- **SEPTICEMIA**
- **CARDIAC FAILURE**
- **HEMORRHAGE**
- **NEUROGENIC SHOCK**

Hypovolemia
- **HEMORRHAGE**
- **GASTROINTESTINAL FLUID LOSS**
- **HYPOPROTEINEMIA**
- **ADRENAL FAILURE**
- **BURNS**

Severe Hypertension
- **MALIGNANT HYPERTENSION**

Hypoxemia
- **CARDIAC FAILURE**
- **RESPIRATORY FAILURE**
- **SERVE ANEMIA**

Hypoglycemia
Renal artery occlusion

Renal

Intrinsic renal parenchymal injury:

Glomerulonephritis
- **POSTSTREPTOCOCCAL GLOMERULONEPHTITIS**
- **MEMBRANOPROLIFERATIVE GLOMERULONEPHRITIS**
- **LUPUS NEPHRITIS**
- **HENOCH-SCHOLEIN PURPURA**
- **HEREDITARY NEPHRITIS**

Nephrotoxicity
- **HEAVY METALS**
- **NEPHROTOXIC CHEMICALS AND DRUGS**
- **HEMOGLOBIN/MYOGLOBIN-URIA**
- **SHOCK**
- **ACUTE TUBULAR ISCHEMIA**

Intravascular coagulation
- **HEMOLYTIC-UREMIC SYNDROME**
- **DISSEMINATED INTRAVASCULAR COAGULATION**
- **CORTICAL NECROSIS**
- **RENAL VEIN THROMBOSIS**

Developmental abnormalities
- **CYSTIC KIDNEYS**
- **HYPOPLASTIC/DYSPLASTIC KIDNEYS**

Postrenal

Obstruction of urine flow from the kidneys:
- **URIC ACID NEPHROPATHY**
- **LITHIASES**
- **EXTRINSIC TUMORS**
- **VESICOURETERAL REFLUX**
- **STRUCTURAL ABNORMALITIES**

Disease Profiles

CONGENITAL ANOMALITIES ASSOCIATED WITH RENAL DISEASE
Cystic Diseases
    POLYCYSTIC DISEASE
        Autosomal recessive form (infantile)
        Autosomal dominant form (adult)
    MEDULLARY CYSTIC DISEASE (NEPHRONOPHTHISIS)
        Autosomal recessive form (juvenile)
        Autosomal dominant form (Adult)
    HEREDITARY AND FAMILIAL CYSTIC DYSPLASIA
        Congenital nephrosis
        "Finnish" disease
Dysplastic Renal Diseases
    RENAL APLASIA
    RENAL HYPOPLASIA
    MULTICYSTIC RENAL DYSPLASIA
    FAMILIAL AND HEREDITARY RENAL DYSPLASIA
    OLIGOMEGANEPHRONIA
Hereditary Diseases Associated with Nephritis
    HEREDITARY NEPHRITIS WITH DEAFNESS AND OCULAR DEFECTS
     (ALPORT SYNDROME)
    NAIL-PATELLA SYNDROME
    FAMILIAL HYPERPROLINEMIA
    HEREDITARY NEPHROTIC SYNDROME
    HEREDITARY OSTEOLYSIS WITH NEPHROPATHY
    HEREDITARY NEPHRITIS WITH THORACIC ASPHYXIANT DYSTROPHY
     SYNDROME
Hereditary Diseases Associated with Intrarenal Deposition of Metabolites
    ANGIOKERATOME CORPORIS DIFFUSUM (FABRY'S DISEASE)
    HEREDOPATHIA ATATICA POLYNEURITIFORMIS (REFSUM DISEASE)
    Various storage diseases
        G$_{M1}$ MONOSIALOGANGLILSIDOSIS
        HURLER SYNDROME
        NIEMAN-PICK DISEASE
        FAMILIAL METACHROMATIC LEUKODYSTROPHY
        GLYCOGENOSIS TYPE I (VON GIERKE'S DISEASE)
        GLYCOGENOSIS TYPE II (POMPE'S DISEASE)
    Hereditary amyloidosis
        FAMILIAL MEDITERRANEAN FEVER
        HEREDOFAMILIAL URTICARIA WITH DEAFNESS AND
         NEUROPATHY
        PRIMARY FAMILIAL AMYLOIDOSIS WITH POLYNEUROPATHY
    Hereditary Renal Diseases Associated With Tubular Transport Defects
        HARTNUP DISEASE
        IMMUNOGLYCINUIA
        FANCONI'S SYNDROME
        OCULOCEREBRORENAL SYNDROME OF LOWE
        CYSTINOSIS
        WILSON'S DISEASE
        GALACTOSEMIA
        HEREDITARY FRUCTOSE INTOLERANCE
        RENAL TUBULAR ACIDOSIS
        HEREDITARY TYROSINEMIA
        RENAL GLYCOSURIA
        VITAMIN D-RESISTANT RICKETS
        PSEUDOHYPOPARATHYROIDISM
        VASOPRESSIN-RESISTANT DIABETES INSIPIDUS
        HYPOURICEMIA
    Hereditary Diseases Associated with Lithiasis
        IDIOPATHIC HYPERCALCURIA
        HYPEROXALURIA
        $_L$-GLYCERIC ACIDURIA
        XANTHINURIA

XANTHINURIA
LESCH-NYHAN SYNDROME
GOUT
FAMILIAL HYPERPARATHYROIDISM
CYSTINURIA
GLYCINURIA

Miscellaneous

HEREDITARY INTESTINAL VITAMIN B_{12} MALADSORPTION
TOTAL AND PARTIAL LIPODYSTROPHY
SICKLE CELL ANEMIA
BARTTER'S SYNDROME

Modified from Gary M. Lum, MD, in Current Pediatric Diagnosis and Treatment, 10/e, (Hathaway, WE, et al. editors), Appleton & Lange, Norwalk, CT, 1991

Glomerular Disorders

Glomerular injury results in two distinct types of functional lesions: inflammatory and non-inflammatory. Non inflammatory glomerular lesions result in protein leakage through the injured filtering interface. These are refered to as nephrotic lesions. In uncomplicated cases, they do not compromise the GFR. Therefore, fluid retention, hypertension, and elevated BUN/Cr are not expected. The prototype of such lesions is seen in the idiopathic nephrotic syndrome of childhood. In inflammatory lesions (nephritic lesions) eroded areas allow loss of particles as large as RBC's, however, the swollen glomeruli decrease the total filtering surface available and cause fluid retention, hypertension and decreased GFR, as well as hematuria. Post streptococcal glomerulonephritis is the protypical inflammatory glomerular lesion. Many glomerular disorders have compontents of both nephrotic and nephritic lesions.

IDIOPATHIC NEPHROTIC SYNDROME OF CHILDHOOD

Most common cause of nephrotic syndrome in children

Alternate terminology
Nil lesion nephrotic syndrome, minimal lesion nephrotic syndrome, lipoid nephrosis of childhood

Etiology
May be an abnormality of a thymic T-cell lymphocytic function resulting in increased permeability of glomerular filtering surfaces.

Pathophysiologic abnormality
Urinary protein loss > 40mg/M^2/hour

Predisposing conditions
male (2:1), age 2-6 years, viral URI

Symptoms
anorexia, abdominal pain, diarrhea, lethergy

Physical findings
edema

Laboratory findings
proteinuria, hypoalbuminemia, hyperlipidemia, Normal C3, BUN, Cr; no hematuria, or RBC casts

Chronologic sequence of manifestations
Proteinuria --> hypoalbuminemia --> edema (periorbital, then dependent, then generalized)

Potential complications
Infections: peritonitis (S.Pneumonia most common)
pneumonia, sepsis, cellulitis, UTI.
Vascular thrombosis, Steriod induced cataracts

Differential diagnosis
Focal segmental glomerulosclerosis, Mesangial proliferative glomerulonephritis

Diagnostic plan
Urine: timed protein excretion, complete urinalyisis
Serum: BUN, Cr, electryoltes, C3, lipid profile, total protein/albumin

Therapeutic plan
Prednisone 2mg/kg/day until proteinuria resolves or 4-6 weeks; then taper.

Prognosis
Good, if steriod responsive. 95% with minimal change disease respond to corticosteroids. If they do not, misdiagnoses must be considered. Relapses may occur with URI's and require retreatment.

FOCAL SEGMENTAL GLOMERULOSCLEROSIS
Initially may be indistinguishable from minimal-change disease. Only 20% with this morphologic lesion respond to corticosteriods. The reaminder progress to end stage renal disease, and, the disease recurs in transplanted kidneys.

MESANGIAL PROLIFERATIVE GLOMERULONEPHRITIS
Also called IgM Nephropathy
Has features of both minimal-change disease and focal segmental glomerulosclerosis. About 50% respond to corticosteriods, the others progress to end stage renal disease.

HEMOLYTIC-UREMIC SYNDROME
Most common cause of acute renal failure in infants and children

Etiology
Has been associated with bacterial (especially E. Coli [O157:H7]), as well as viral gastrointestinal infections.

Pathophysiologic abnormality
Renal vascular endothelial injury results from platelet deposition and consumption. Red cells are broken up as they pass through the fibrin strands, and renal perfusion is compromised. The result is the characteristic triad of azotemia, thrombocytopenia, and microangiopathic hemolytic anemia

Symptoms
fever, vomiting, diarrhea (often bloody), irratability, altered sensorium, olguria

Physical findings
edema, pallor, petechiae, hepatosplenomegaly

Laboratory findings
Elevated BUN/Cr, anemia, elevated reticulocyte count, elevated bilirubin, leukocytosis, thrombocytopenia, negative Coombs test, helment/burr cells on periphreal smear, normal C3

Chronologic sequence of manifestations
gastroenteritis signs and symptoms followed by 7 to 10 days improvement, then acute onset of renal failure and anemia

Potential complications
problems due to acute renal failure and diffuse vasculitis and/or intravascular thrombosis.

Differential diagnosis
Bilateral renal vein thrombosis, lupus nephritis,

acute glomerulonephritis
Therapeutic plan
Treatment of the acute renal failure.
Plasmaphoresis is advocated by some.
Prognosis
Recovery of renal function has occured after 2 or more weeks of anuria. Hypertension, chronic renal failure and CVA's or other intravascular thrombotic phenomenae are worrisome potential late sequelae.

POSTSTREPTOCOCCAL GLOMERULONEPHRITIS
Competes with IgA nephropathy as the most common cause of gross hematuria in children
Etiology
Nephritogenic strains of group A beta-hemolytic streptococci
Pathophysiologic abnormality
Inflammatory glomerular lesions causing decreased GFR and fluid retention
Predisposing conditions
Streptococcal pharyngitis or impetigo
Symptoms
tea-colored urine, oliguria, lethargy, maliase,abdominal pain, flank pain, fever,
Physical findings
edema, hypertension, fluid overload
Laboratory findings
urine: RBC casts, hematuria, proteinuria, WBC's.
serum: low C3 complement, positive Streptozyme test, elevated ASO titer (post pharyngitis; not impetigo), elevated BUN/Cr, normal proteins,
Chronologic sequence of manifestations
Streptococcal infection, then renal insult. The C3 returns to normal within 8 weeks
Potential complications
renal failure with fluid overload, hypertension, uremia
Differential diagnosis
other causes of hematuria
Diagnostic plan
monitor BP, urinalysis, C3 complement, BUN/Cr, CBC, Streptozyme test, Protein
Therapeutic plan
sodium and fluid restriction, loop diuretics, antihypertensives, if BP elevated
Prognosis
95% recover completely. Morbidity may result from uncontrolled hypertension.

POSTINFECTIOUS NON-STREPTOCOCCAL GLOMERULONEPHRITIS
Other causes of acute infection-mediated glomerulonephritis include:
Bacterial: staphlococcal (shunt nephritis);
Viral: hepatitis B, infectious mononucleosis, CMV infections;
Fungal: histoplasmosis;
Parasitic: toxoplasmosis, falciparum malaria

MEMBRANOPROLIFERATIVE GLOMERULONEPHRITIS
Most common cause of chronic glomerulonephritis in older children and adults
Also called mesangiocapillary GMN. Once differientiated from other causes of chronic GMN by the finding of decreased C3, but now distinguished by 3 histologic subtypes:

Type I
Type II
Type III
Presents in the 2nd decade of life with proteinuria and hematuria. Most develop nephrotic syndrome. Many progress to end stage renal disease. Renal biopsy is required for the diagnosis since hypocomplementemia does not always occur.

MEMBRANOUS GLOMERULOPATHY
Most common cause of nephrotic syndrome in adults
Clinical manifestations are similar to membranoproliferative GMN except the C3 is normal, and most cases in children resolve spontaneous;y.

RAPIDLY PROGRESSIVE GOLMERULONEPHRITIS
Also called diffuse crescentic GMN. If the typical glomerular crescents are not due to poststreptococcal, membranoproliferative, anaphylactoid purpura, lupus or Goodpasture disease progression to end stage renal disease can be expected within months of onset. C3 is normal. Diagnosis is made by renal biopsy.

HEREDITARY GLOMERULONEPHRITIS
The most commom form is Alport's syndrome which presents around school age with asymptomatic hematuria followed by development of proteinuria. Many have hypertension, which may be severe, and one- third have sensorineural hearling loss. Eye problems also occur in 15% of patients.

LUPUS NEPHRITIS
Nephritis is a common manifestation of lupus erythematosus in childhood
Adolescent females are most commonly affected.Normalization of C3 reflects effective immunosuppressive therapy. The renal injury may progress to end stage renal disease. It is a disease characterized by remissions and relapses as it progresses. Complications may occur both from the disease and from the therapy it requires.

IgA NEPHROPATHY
Alternate terminology
Berger's nephropathy
Pathogenesis
IgA deposition on glomerular basement membranes
Predisposing conditions
URI's, male sex
Laboratory findings
Normal C3, micorscopic and gross hematuria, non-nephrotic proteinuria
Potential complications
20% develop hypertension, nephrotic syndrome, and eventual renal failure. The nephropathy recurs in transplanted kidneys.

HENOCH-SCHONLEIN PURPURA GLOMERULONEPHRITIS
Alternate terminology
Anaphylactoid purpura GMN
Pathophysiologic abnormality
Small vessel vasculitis, which can cause decreased

GFR
Symptoms
abdominal pain, arthralgia
Physical findings
urticarial and/or purpuric rash on buttocks and lower extemeties, joint effusions
Laboratory findings
hematuria, proteinuria, normal C3 and platelets
Chronologic sequence of manifestations
Urticarial rash progresses to palpable purpuric lesions. Abdominal pain which promptly resolves following institution of corticosteroid therapy is typical
Potential complications
Intussusception, bowel perforation.
Severe renal involvement is rare.
Prognosis
When severe renal involvement occurs, it is unresponsive to treatment.

SICKLE CELL NEPHROPATHY
The intital defect is usually in concentrating ability of the tubules. Renal involvement may progress to include episodic hematuria and a nephrotic syndrome.

Juxtaglomerular Disorders

Histologically demonstratable juxtaglorerular disorders are extremely rare, but the disorders in its differential are not. Urine chloride is helpful since those disorders associated with hypovolemia have low urine chloride levels.

BARTTER SYNDROME
Pathology
Generalized hyperplasia of the juxtaglomerular apparatus
Pathophysiologic abnormality
A defect in chloride readsorbtion in the ascending loop of Henle results in urinary potassium wasting when excess NaCl presents to the distal tubule and is readsorbed in exchange for potassium. Hypokalemia stimulates prostaglandin and renin synthesis. The elevated prostaglandin contributes to a defect in platelet aggregation, and the elevated renin stimulates aldosterone production which exacerbates the hypokalemia.
Symptoms
muscle weakness, polyuria, constipation, carpo-pedal spasms
Physical findings
dehydration, growth failure, normal blood pressure
Laboratory findings
severe hypokalemia, defective platelet aggregation, hypochloremic metabolic alkalosis, elevated renin, elevated aldosterone, elevated prostaglandin E_2, elevated urine potassium, elevated urine chloride
Differential diagnosis
licorice abuse, pyelonephritis, diabetes insipidus, chronic vomiting, chronic diarrhea, laxative abuse, diuretic use

Interstitial Disorders

ACUTE INTERSTITIAL NEPHRITIS
A disorder of unknown etilolgy characterized by interstitial inflammation and edema. Most often due to drug therapy and in such cases may be a hypersensitivity reaction. It is also seen in association with infections and other disorders, including renal transplant rejection. Staining of the urinary sediment for eosinophils may be helpful in identifying this entity. Diagnosis is made by renal biopsy.

CHRONIC INTERSITITAL NEPHRITIS
Once the interstitial edema of acute interstitial nephritis is replaced by fibrosis, the condition is progressive and end-stage renal failure ensues.

Tubular Disorders

RENAL TUBULAR ACIDOSIS
A heterogeneous group of disorders, all of which have hyperchloremic metabolic acidosis, and tubular dysfunction. Renal failure is not an expected component of this group of disorders.

RENAL TUBULAR ACIDOSIS TYPE I
Alternate terminology
Distal renal tubular acidosis
Etiology
May be primary or secondary to obstructive uropathy, pyelonephritis, sickle cell nephropathy, lupus nephritis, medullary sponge kidney, renal transplant rejection, or toxins
Pathophysiologic abnormality
Defective hydrogen ion secretion in the distal tubule, which results in up to 15% of the filtered sodium bicarbonate load being lost in the urine.
Symptoms
failure to thrive, anorexia, vomiting
Physical findings
dehydration
Laboratory findings
hyperchloremic metabolic acidosis, mild hypokalemia, alkaline urine
Potential complications
hypercalcuria, nephrocalcinosis, renal stones
Therapeutic plan
2-3 meq/kg/24hr $NaHCO_3$ is theraputic and distinguishes this from the proximal type which requires > 10 meq/kg/24hr.
Prognosis
good if renal injury can be avoided

RENAL TUBULAR ACIDOSIS TYPE II
Alternate terminology
Proximal renal tubular acidosis
Etiology
May be primary, a component of Fanconi

syndrome, or due to tubular immaturity in premature infants

Pathophysiologic abnormality

Lowered renal threshold for bicarbonate readsorption in the proximal tubule. If serum acidosis drops below this threshold, the urine becomes acidic.

Laboratory findings

hyperchloremic metabolic acidosis, hypokalemia

Potential complications

rarely nephrocalcinosis

Therapeutic plan

high (> 5 meq/kg/24hr) doses of bicarbonate

Prognosis

Excellent if isolated lesion, otherwise dependent on underlying disorder.

RENAL TUBULAR ACIDOSIS TYPE III

Type I with an associated bicarbonate tubular leak

RENAL TUBULAR ACIDOSIS TYPE IV

Alternate terminology

Mineralocorticoid deficiency RTA

Etiology

Disorders with:

decreased aldosterone and elevated renin:

Adrenal failure, Congenital adrenal hyperplasia, Primary hypoaldosteronism

decreased aldosterone and decreased renin:

pyelonephritis, interstitial nephritis, obstructive lesions, nephrosclerosis, diabetes mellitus

increased aldosterone and increased renin

Pseudohypoaldosteronism

DIFFUSE PROXIMAL RENAL TUBULAR DYSFUNCTION

Alternate terminology

Fanconi syndrome

Etiology

Inherited disorders: Cystinosis, Lowe syndrome, Glactosemia, Tyrosinemia, Heriditary fructose intolerance, Glycogen storage disease type I, Wilson disease, Medullary cystic disease

Systemic disorders: Rubella syndrome, Amyloidosis, Sjogren syndrome

Toxins: heavy metals, outdated tetracycline, Lindane, hyperparathyroidism, interstitial nephritis

Pathophysiologic abnormality

Defect in proximal tubular function

Laboratory findings

Hyperchloremic metabolic acidosis, glycosuria, aminoaciduria, depressed tubular readsorption of phosphate

Prognosis

Dependent on the underlying disorder

NEPHROGENIC DIABETES INSIPIDUS

Etiology

Primary form is X-linked recessive and completely expressed and only partly in females.

All forms are diagnosed by lack of response to vasopressin.

Urologic Disorders

If the following are considered possibilities in the differential diagnosis of causes of azotemia in children, imaging studies may be indicated.

HYPRONEPHROSIS
UROLITHIASIS
NEUROGENIC BLADDER
URETHRAL STENOSIS
POSTERIOR URETHREAL VALVES

Should always be considered in the differential of causes of azotemia in male infants.

HYPOSPADIAS

Avoid circumscisions, since the foreskin is used in repair of the lesion.

CRYPTORCHIDISM

Should be surgically corrected (orchiopexy) by age 2 years.

TESTICULAR TORSION

A true surgical emergency as delayed correction can lead to loss of the testicle.

A. Eugene Osburn

Developmental Considerations

Osmolality

This is the mechanism which governs distribution of body fluids across the compartments' semipermeable membranes. The normal osmolality is 285 mosm/L.

Fluid Spaces

Total body water

70-75% of total body weight in the newborn. After the postnatal diuresis, it is 65% and remains constant until puberty when it decreases to 55-60%. About 2/3 of the TBW is intracellular and the rest extracellular fluid.

Extracellular Fluid

Sodium is the predominant cation of the ECF. It is present in a concentration of 140 mEq/L. ECF contains only 4 mEq/L of potassium. Regulation of the ECF volume is through the interaction of the antidiuretic hormone (ADH), thirst and the renin-angiotensin-aldolsterone axis. Distribution of fluid between the two compartments of the ECF (**Plasma Fluid** and **Interstitial Fluid**) is regulated primarily by the oncotic pressure of plasma proteins. The clinical signs of dehydration are a reflection of changes in the ECF volume.

Intracellular Fluid

Potassium is the major cation in the ICF. Its concentration there is around 160 mEq/L.

Daily Fluid Requirements

Body Weight (kg)	Maintenance water required
Up to 10	100 cc/kg
11-20	1000cc +
	50 cc/kg for each kg over 10 kg
Above 20	1500 cc/kg +
	20 cc/kg for each kg over 20 kg

Daily Electrolyte Requirements

Cation	Maintenance Requirement
Sodium	3 mEq/kg/24 hours
Potassium	2 mEq/kg/24 hours

Diagnostic Modalities

Clinical assessment of degree of dehydration			
Parameter	Mild (<5%)	Moderate (10%)	Severe (15%)
Skin color	Pink	Acrocyanosis	Mottled
Tears	Present	Reduced	Absent
Mucous Membrane	Normal	Dry	Parched
Eyeball	Normal	Depressed	Sunken
Fontanelle	Normal	Depressed	Sunken
Level of Consciousness	Alert	Lethargic	Obtunded
Pulse Rate	Upper Normal	Increased	Markedly increased
Capillary Refill	Upper Normal	Definately Prolonged	Markedly Prolonged
Blood Pressure	Normal	Orthostatic Hypotension	Recumbent Hypotension
BUN	Normal	Elevated	Very high
Arterial pH	7.40-7.30	7.30-7.00	< 7.10
Urine Volume	Small	Oliguria	Oliguria/anuria
Specific gravity	<1.020	> 1.030	> 1.035

Anion Gap

The anion gap reflects the amount of organic acids present in the serum. It can be calculated by the formula:

$$\text{Anion gap} = (Na^+ + K^+) - (Cl^- + HCO_3^-) = 8 \text{ to } 12 \text{ mEq/L}$$

Osmolar Gap

The difference between measured osmolality and calculated osmolality.
The expected osmolality can be calculated by the formula:

$$\text{Plasma osmolality} = 2 \times (Na^+) + \frac{\text{Glucose}}{18} + \frac{\text{BUN}}{2.8}$$

GENERAL ACID-BASE RULES OF THUMB

A 1 mmHg increase in $PaCO_2$ causes a 0.01 decrease in pH.
A 1 mEq/L decrease in HCO_3 causes a 0.02 decrease in pH.
A 0.1 increase in pH causes a 0.5 mEq/L decrease in K^+.
A 0.1 increase in pH shifts the oxygen dissociation curve to the left enough to decrease O_2 release to tissues by 10%.

Pathophysiologic Manifestations

Causes of hypernatremia

Hypernatremia associated with decreased ECF
Due to extrarenal water losses (urine Na < 10 meq/L)
skin losses
respiratory losses
gastrointestinal losses
severe burns
Thyrotoxicosis
Due to renal water losses (urine Na > 40 meq/L)
diuretics
renal disease
relief of urinary obstruction
osmoreceptor failure
Hypernatremia associated with normal ECF
Impaired thirst
Nonrenal water losses
Renal water losses
Hypernatremia associated with increased ECF
Iatrogenic saline excess
Mineralocorticoid excess
hyperaldosteronism
Cushings disease
congenital adrenal hyperplasia
exogenous corticosteroids

Causes of hyponatremia

Hyponatremia associated with decreased ECF

Due to extrarenal sodium losses (urine Na < 20 meq/L)
- Sweating
- Vomiting/Diarrhea
- Burn fluid loss
- Peritonitis
- Pancreatitis

Due to renal sodium losses (urine Na > 40 meq/L)
- Aldosterone deficiency
- Salt losing nephropathy
- Renal tubular diuritics
- Osmotic diuretics

Hyponatremia associated with normal ECF

[Normal BUN, no edema]

Inappropriate ADH secretion (SIADH)

"Appropriate" excess ADH secretion
- Pain, physical/emotional stress
- Myxedema

Without excess ADH secretion
- Water intoxication
  - Iatrogenic water overload
  - Psychogenic polydispia
- Sick cell (reset osmostat) syndrome

Hyponatremia associated with increased ECF

Decreased GFR and abnormal tubules (oliguria, urine sodium > 40 meq/L)
- Renal failure

Decreased GFR with normal tubules (oliguria, urine sodium < 20 meq/L)

[decreased vascular volume and/or cardiac output]
- Cardiac failure
- Hepatic failure
- Nephrotic syndrome

Factitious Hyponatremia
- Hyperglycemia
- Hyperlipidemia
- Hyperproteinemia

Since glucose remains extracellular in hyperglycemia, it draws intracellular water into the extracellular space and factitiously dilutes the measured sodium there. The true serum sodium concentration in hyperglycemia can be calculated by assuming the sodium is diluted 1.6 to 1.8 mEq/L for each 100 mg/dl the glucose is above its normal 100 mg/dl.

Fluid and Electrolyte Treatment Guidelines

Maintenance Fluids

Maintenance fluids can be provided by using D_5W 1/4 NS plus 20-30 mEq/L KCl. The infusion rate can be calculated using the expected 24 hour fluid volume requirement guidelines given above, or can be directly calculated as an hourly rate by the following:

Hourly Maintenance Fluid Rate

0 to 10 kg: 4 cc/kg/hr

11 to 20 kg: 40 cc/hr +
2 cc/kg/hr for each kg > 10

> 20 kg: 60 cc/kg/hr +
1 cc/kg/hr for each kg > 20

Hypernatremia

Hypernatremia with edema and a normal BUN (unless in shock) is due to salt poisoning and requires urgent dialysis.

The serum soduim in hypernatremic dehydration must be replaced slowly, over 48 hours, to avoid too rapid osmolar shifts of water into brain cells with resulting cerebral edema. For the same reason, the replacement fluid should be at least 1/4 Normal Saline, not dextrose in water alone.

The degree of dehydration estimated from clinical signs of dehydration relies on findings reflecting the extracellular fluid volume. In hypernatremic dehydration the amount of fluid loss is often underestimated because the fluid shift from the intracellular space in hypertonic dehydration delays clinical manifestations of the amount of TBW lost. The acutal water deficit in hypernatremic dehydration can be estimated by:

Normal total body water (TBW) = 0.6 X normal wt (kg)

$$\frac{\text{Normal Na}}{\text{Measured Na}} \times \text{TBW} = \text{current TBW}$$

Fluid deficit = Normal TBW - current TBW

Hyponatremia

Symptomatic hyponatremia rarely occurs unless the serum Na is less than 120 mEq/L, and symptoms such as seizures are more the result of the rapidity of fall in sodium concentration than the level reached.

A key to assessing the approach to treatment of hyponatremia is the BUN.

Hyponatremia with a normal BUN is due either to inappropriate ADH secretion or water intoxication and the treatment of either of these conditions is water restriction, not fluid replacement, unless the hyponatremia is symptomatic.

Symptomatic hyponatremia is best treated with hypertonic saline (3%). The volume required to raise the serum Na above 120 mEq/L can be calculated by the formula:

(Desired Na [i.e. 120 mEq/L] - measured Na) X 0.6 X wt (kg) = mEq Na required.

3% saline contains 0.5 mEq Na/cc.

Hyperkalemia

Physiologically significant hyperkalemia is reflected in the EKG. The earliest change in the EKG is a tenting or peaking of the T waves.

Treatement of hyperkalemia includes calcium gluconate (calcium chloride can worsen acidosis usually present in hyperkalemic conditions), sodium bicarbonate, insulin and glucose, and a cation exchange resin (Kayexalate). These are listed in descending order of rapidity on onset of action and ascending order of duration of action. Dialysis may be needed for situations not adequately controlled by the preceeding temporary measures.

Hypokalemia

Total body potassium deficits are not necessarily reflected in serum potassium values. A urine potassium of < 20 mEq/L, however, reflectes the normal kidney's effort to conserve the potassium presented to its tubules. Thus, urine potassium should guide replacement of total body potassium deficits.

Physiologically significant hypokalemia is reflected in the EKG with ST segment depression, T wave amplitude reduction and U waves.

Except in unusual circumstances, potassium concentration in I.V. fluids should not exceed 40 mEq/L.

Guidelines for treatment of dehydration

	Weight loss per severity			Replacement Fluid	Hours for deficit replacement	
	Mild	Moderate	Severe		1st 1/2	2nd 1/2
Hypotonic dehydration	2%	5%	10%	D$_5$W 3/4 NS	4	20
Isotonic dehydration	5%	10%	15%	D$_5$W 1/2 NS	8	16
Hypertonic dehydration	10%	15%	20%	D$_5$W 1/4 NS	24	24

1. Correct shock with boluses of 20 cc/kg of D$_5$W NS.
   If additional volume expansion is needed use plasminate or albumin
2. Obtain results for BUN, Cr, Na, K, Cl, HCO, and glucose
3. Estimate severity of dehydration.
4. Based on severity estimated and type identified with the electrolyte results, multiply the percent from the above by the body weight and using the composition of fluid from the replacement fluid column replace one half the deficit volume over each of the number of hours depicted.
5. Add KCl in a concentration of 20 - 40 mEq/L to the replacement fluid as soon as adequate urine flow is assured.

The above volumes and concentrations should be added to the daily maintenance fluid reqirement to avoid getting behind from failing to provide ongoing needs.

Theraputic endpoints for treatment of dehydration

GOAL	TIME FRAME
Adequate urine volume	First hour
Urine specific gravity = 1.010	First few hours *
Normal electrolytes	Hours (hyponatremia) to 2 days (Hypernatramia)
Elevated BUN decreased by 1/2	Every 15 - 20 hours
Normal Acid-Base Status	One to three days
Urine potassium > 40 mEq/L	Three to 5 days

* After the urine specific gravity has decreased to 1.010, the infusion rate of fluids can be decreased to maintenance rates since the kidneys will just excrete any excess at that point.

Acid-Base disturbances

A pH of 7.40 is the result of a ratio of HCO_3 to $PaCO_2$ of 20 to 1. Changes in this ratio cause a corresponding change in the pH. This is reflected in the following formula:

$$pH = \frac{HCO_3}{PaCO_2} = \frac{24 \text{ mEq/L}}{40 \text{ mmHg}} = \frac{20}{1} = 7.40$$

(40 mmHg x 0.03 = 1.2 mEq/L)

The $PaCO_2$ is dependent on the minute volume of respiration and can change in minutes. The HCO_3 is regulated by the kidneys and changes take hours to days. Any change in either of these determiners of pH is accompanied by a compensatory change in the other. The results of such changes is depicted in the table that follows:

	HCO_3 mEq/L < 21	HCO_3 mEq/L 21 - 26	HCO_3 mEq/L > 26
$PaCO_2$ mmHg > 45	Combined Metabolic Acidosis and Respiratory Acidosis	Respiratory Acidosis	Mixed Metabolic Alkalosis and Respiratory Acidosis
$PaCO_2$ mmHg 35 - 45	Metabolic Acidosis	NORMAL	Metabolic Alkalosis
$PaCO_2$ mmHg < 35	Mixed Metabolic Acidosis and Respiratory Acidosis	Respiratory Alkalosis	Combined Respiratory Alkalosis and Metabolic Alkalosis

In mixed disorders, the pH reflects which mixed disorder pair is primary and which is secondary since compensation is never complete nor over-compensated. The mechanisms for the compensatory changes are:

Organ effecting the change	Direction of change	Mechanism
	Elevated HCO_3	
KINDEY: HCO_3		HCO_3 generated via acidification of urine
		Must have Na^+ and K^+ available for exchange with HCO_3 to alkalinize urine
	Decreased HCO_3	

$pH = $ --

	Elevated $PaCO_2$	
		Hypoventilation
LUNG: $PaCO_2$		
		Hyperventilation
	Decreased $PaCO_2$	

Expected compensatory changes in primary acid-base disorders

disorder	initial change	compensatory change
Respiratory Acidosis	10 mmHg $PaCO_2$ increase	HCO_3 increases 1 mEq/L (acute) HCO_3 increases 3-4 mEq/L (chronic)
Respiratory Alkalosis	10 mmHg $PaCO_2$ decrease	HCO_3 decreases 1-3 mEq/L (acute) HCO_3 decreases 2-5 mEq/L (chronic)
Metabolic Acidosis	1 mEq/L HCO_3 decrease	$PaCO_2$ decreases 1-1.5 mmHg
Metabolic Alkalosis	1 mEq/L HCO_3 increase	$PaCO_2$ increases 0.5-1 mmHg

In primary metabolic acidosis, the $PaCO_2$ in mmHg should equal the 2 digits to the right of the decimal point of the pH if no other derrangement exists. e.g. a pH of 7.22 corresponds to a $PaCO_2$ of 22 mmHg in pure acute metabolic acidosis without compensatory changes.

Causes of Metabolic Alkalosis

Chloride responsive causes (urine Cl < 10 mEq/L)

Gastrointestinal chloride loss

vomiting

gastric suction

chloride diarrhea

Diuretics

rapid correction of hypercapnia

Cystic Fibrosis

Chloride resistant causes (urine Cl > 20 mEq/L)

Excess mineralcorticoid activity

Hyperaldosteronism

Cushings syndrome

Bartters syndrome

Excess licorice

Severe K depletion

Variable chloride response

Milk-alkali syndrome

Alkali adminstration

Causes of Metabolic Acidosis

Increased loss of bicarbonate or chloride addition (normal anion gap)

Associated with potassium retention (hyperkalemia)

Early uremic acidosis

Renal tubular acidosis type IV

Hyopaldosteronism

Potassium sparing diuretics

Resolving DKA

Early obstructive uropathy

Associated with potassium depletion (hypokalemia)

Acute diarrhea with HCO and Cl losses

Renal tubular acidosis type I

Renal tubular acidosis type II

Dilution acidosis

Increased organic acids (increased anion gap)

A	aspirin, alcohol ketoacidosis
M	methanol
U	uremia
D	diabetic ketoacidosis
P	paraldehyde
I	iron, ibuprofen, isoniazide
L	lactic acidosis
E	ethylene glycol
S	starvation ketoacidosis

Causes of Respiratory Alkalosis

Anxiety/hyperventilation
CNS pathology
      infection, trauma, tumors
Hypoxia
      Mild bronchospasm
      Congestive heart failure
      Pneumonia
      Pulmonary emboli
      Severe anemia
Respiratory center stimulating drugs
      Salicylates
      Catecholamines
Pregnancy
Pain
Fever/sepsis
Hepatic dysfunction
Hyperthyroidism

Causes of Respiratory Acidosis

CNS depression of respiratory drive
      Drug overdose
      CNS lesions
      CNS infections
Pulmonary diseases
      Obstructive pulmonary disease
      Severe bronchospasm
      Pneumonia
      Pulmonary edema
      Smoke inhalation
Mechanical abnormalities
      Airway obstruction
      Foreign body
      croup
      epiglottitis
      retropharyngeal abscess
      laryngeal edema
      aspiration
      Plerual effusion
      Pneumothorax
      Flail chest
      Scoliosis
Neuromuscular abnormalities
      Guillain-Barre syndrome
      Poliomyelitis
      Wernig-Hoffman disease
      Myasthenia gravis
      Botulism
      Tetanus
      Muscular dystrophy
      Severe hypokalemia
      Myxedema

A. Eugene Osburn

Developmental Considerations

Optimal brain growth and development requires structural integrity, adequate nutritional substrates at the appropriate time, absence of toxic and traumatic insults and environmental stimulation. Deficiencies in any of these areas can result in suboptimal neurological development.

The skull grows in response to developing brain tissue. Microcephaly is due to smaller than average brain volume. Lack of skull growth does not cause microcephaly.

Physical brain growth continues until around ten years of age. At birth, the head is 3/4 the adult size. One half the adult size is reached by one year of age. Myelinization of the spinal cord is not completed until two years after birth.

Diagnostic Modalities

Serum electrolytes, glucose, Magnesium and Calcuim
A fingerstick glucose should be done early in evaluation of altered sensorium. Hypoglycemia can cause profound, and if not rapidly enough reversed, permanent CNS changes. Determination of the other electolytes and minerals may detect treatable causes of CNS dysfunction.

Toxicology Screens
A toxicology screen should always be considered in cases in which neurologic changes do not have a obvious explaination. In seizure patients with neurologic changes anticonvulsant levels are indicated.

Lumbar Puncture (LP) and Cerebrospinal Fluid (CSF) analysis
The most common parameters assessed via a LP are: opening pressure, CSF cell count, CSF protein, CSF glucose, Counter Current Immune Electophoresis (CCIE), and gram stain. In uncooperative infants and children, the opening pressure may not be done because of questionable validity. Before performing the LP, one must be sure there is no evidence of significant increased intracranial pressure by noting the absence of papilledema, or, if time and the situation permit, a CT scan of the head. Focal neurologic deficits should especially raise the question of significant incracranial mass effect.

Normal CSF values

Age	Opening Pressure	Glucose	Protein	Cells Polys	Lymphs	RBCs
Newborn	70- 180 mm H$_2$O	50-80 mg/dl	150 mg/dl	< 8	< 30	< 50
3 months		(2/3 of blood	< 65 mg/dl	< 3	< 15	<30
> 6 months	70 - 150	glucose)	10 - 40 mg/dl	0	< 5	<5

Electroencephalography (EEG)

The electroencephalogram is being replaced by MRI, evoked potentials, CT scans, and regional blood flow studies as both a diagnostic and prognostic tool in many of the neurological conditions it was relied on before the availability of these modalities. It is still useful to confirm, classify the type of seizure, and monitor response to anticonvulsant therapy in seizure disorders.

Evoked Potentials

Computer enhanced averaging of responses to cortical auditory, visual, or somatosensory evoked responses can be used by skilled interpreters to arrive at clinical interpretions of brain functional interegerty with fairly reproducible results. They are becoming an extremely useful adjunct to the neurologic exam.

CT Scan of the head

The CT scan can reveal structural abnormalities, midline shifts from mass lesions, acute and chronic bleeds, tumors and cerebral edema.

A CT without contrast media is indicated in suspected acute CNS bleeds. It may not, however, detect chronic subdural hematomas if the clot has organized sufficiently to be of similar density to surrounding brain tissue.

A CT with contrast media is needed to best delineate vascularized tumors, A-V malformations and chronic subdural clots. Contrast media should not be used if the patient has evidence of decreased GFR (elevated BUN/Cr), however, as its use in that situation can result in renal shutdown.

Magnetic resonance imaging (MRI)

The MRI is a noninvasive technique that provides more detailed delineation of white and gray matter of the brain and can provide information about not only structural abnormalities, but histological and biochemical information as well. It can not detect calcified lesions, however, and it requires much longer immobilization. It usually requires sedation in children.

Pathophysiologic Manifestations

Common causes of altered mental status in children by age group

Infant	Child	Adolescent
Birth asphyxia	Ingestion	Ingestion
Infection	Infection	Intentional
Inborn Error of	Intussusception	Trauma
Metabolism	Seizure	Drug/alcohol abuse
Abuse	Abuse	
Metabolic disorders		

Causes of seizures by age group

First day of life

Hypoxia   Hyperglycemia
Drugs   Hypoglycemia
Trauma   Pyridoxine deficiency
Infection

Day 2-3 of life

Infection   Developmental malformation
Drug withdrawal   Intracranial hemorrhage
Hypoglycemia   Inborn Error of metabolism
Hypocalcemia   Hyponatremia/hypernatremia

One week to six months of life

Infection   Developmental malformation
Hypocalcemia   Drug withdrawal
Hyperphosphatemia   Inborn Error of Metabolism
Hyponatremia

Six month to 3 years of age

Febrile seizures   Trauma
Birth injury   Metabolic disorder
Infection   Cerebral degenerative disease
Toxins

Over 3 years of age

Idiopathic   Trauma
Infection   Cerebral degenerative disease

Differentiating upper motor neuron from lower motor unit lesions

Finding	Upper motor neuron	Motor unit
Posture	arm flexed, leg extended	flaccid
Reflexes	Increased	Decreased or absent
Tone	Increased	Decreased
Fasciculations	Absent	Present
Atrophy	Absent or mimimal	Present
Muscles affected	Muscle groups	Individual muscles or groups

Upper motor neuron: the corticospinal tract and its motor neurons
Motor unit: includes lower motor neruon (the anterior horn cells, motor nerves, and periphreal motor nerves), neuromuscular junction and muscles.

Diseases of the lower motor unit in infants and children

Anterior Horn Cell
>   **Spinal muscular atrophy (Werdig-Hoffman disease)**
>   **Poliomyelitis**

Periphreal Nerve
>   **Guillian-Barre syndrome**
>   **Tick paralysis**

Neuromuscular Junction
>   **Myasthenia gravis**
>   **Botulism**

Muscle
>   **Muscle Dystrophy**
>>   **Duchene**
>>   **Becker**
>>   **Limb girlde**
>>   **Facioscapulohumeral**
>>   **Myotonic**
>>   **Congenital**

Metabolic, Endocrine, and Mineral
>   **Glycogen Storage disease type II (Pmmpe disease)**
>   **Carnitine Metabolism abnormalities**
>   **Mitrochondrial abnormalities**
>   **Thyroid excess or deficiency**
>   **Cortisol excess or deficiency**
>   **Hyperparathyroidism; calcium excess**
>   **Potassium excess or deficiency**

A. Eugene Osburn

Developmental Considerations

Many skeletal deformities in infancy are due to positional pressures and forces in utero and will resolve spontaneously without treatment.

Foot deformities which can be manipulated back to a normal position will generally resolve spontaneously without corrective devices or appliances.

Corrective shoes do not correct and are an unnecessary expense for parents.

Varum refers to angulation of a bone toward the midline; thus, genu varus means bowleg, since the leg distal to the knee bends toward the midline

Valgum refers to angulation of the bone distal to a joint away from the midline; thus, genu valgum refers to knock knee. (remember, the bottom of the L in valgum bends out from the midline)

Genu varum is normal from infancy until about 3 years of life. Then the normal child commonly has genu valum until about 8 years of age.

Flatfeet are normal in infants.

A septic hip is an orthopedic emergency. Delay in diagnosis and effective treatment can result in permenant loss of the joint.

Puncture wounds of the soles of the feet (especially through dirty tennis shoes) are prone to Pseudomonas aerugonsa osteomyelitis.

Ligaments around joints are stronger than epiphyseal plates in children. Be wary of diagnosing sprains in joints that still have growth plates. It is usually the epiphysis that gives.

Growing pains occur between the age of 5 and 12 years while children are growing. They usually involve the legs, follow strenuous day time activity and do not disturb normal sleep. They are benign.

Pathophysiologic Manifestations

Causes of arthritis and joint pain in children

Condition	Key features
Congenital disorders	
Sickle cell disease	Dactylitis may be first manifestation of the disease in the infant
Hemophilia	Males only. Purpuric lesions are often palpable in the infant.
Trauma	
Sprain	Be wary of sprains in ligaments attached to and around growth plated. It may be a fracture instead.
Fracture	
Tendonitis	
Infections	
Toxic synovitis	Rule out septic joint and osteomyelitis.
Septic Joint	
Viral infections	
Lyme disease	Erythema chronicum migrans rash
Osteomyelitis	
Autoimmune disorders	
Rheumatic fever	Migratory polyarthritis; usually large joints
Juvenile rheumatoid arthritis	Systemic onset: fever > 39.4 for > 2 weeks
	No or low grade fever with:
	> 4 joints: pauciarticular
	< 5 joints: polyarticular
Systemic lupus erythematosis	Typically an arthralgia, not arthritis.
Seurm sickness	Drug reactions are a common cause.
Inflammatory bowel disease	
Henoch-Schonlein purpura	Purpura lesions may be palpable. Indurated antioedema may be present. Abdominal pain responds to corticosteroids.
Neoplastic disorders	
Ewing's sarcoma	
Osteogenic sarcoma	
Leukemia	
Neuroblastoma	

Salter-Harris fracture classification

Type I
Fracture extends through
the epiphyseal plate

Type II
includes a triangular
segment of the
metaphysis

Type III
From the joint
surface to the
epiphyseal plate

Type IV
As in type III
but includes also
adjacent metaphyssis

Type V
Crush injury of
the epiphysis

Common Regional Musculoskeletal Problems

General musculoskeletal disorders

Congenital amputations

May be due to amniotic bands, teratogens, or rarely hereditary defects. Most are spontaneous and are not expected to recur in offspring.

Achondroplasia (Classic Chondrodystrophy)

The limbs are short, with the humerus and femur proportionally shorter than the radius and tibia. Varum deformities are usual. Moderate hydrocephalus, lumbar lordosis, short stubby digits, restriction of motion of major joints are common. Mentality and sexual function are normal. The condition is usually familial.

Osteopetrosis (Albers-Schonberg Disease; Marble Bone Disease)

Characterized by pathologic fractures, myelophthistic anemia, splenomegaly, dwarfing, pigeon breast, square head, facial paralysis, auditory and visual distrubances. Calicification of soft tissues may occur. It is familial. The findings appear at any age.

Rickets

Rickets occurs when growing bone is inadequately mineralized and softens. The excessive osteoid formation causes widening of the metaphyses which results in the characteristic delay in linear growth, widening of wrists and knees, bowing of the legs and prominant costochondral junctions (rachitic rosary). Inadequate dietary vitamin D, lack of adsorption of vitamin D due to fat maladsorption, or defects in vitamin D in the liver or kidney can all cause rickets.

Osteochondrodystrophy (Morquio's Disease)

A result of abnormal deposition of mucopolysaccharides, it is characterized by shortening of the spine, scolosis, kyphosis, pigeon breast, hepatosplenomegaly and corneal clouding. The child appears normal at birth and develops the deformities between 1 and 4 years of age. The condition is an autosomal recessive when familial.

Chondroectodermal dysplasia (Ellis-Van Creveld Syndrome)

Mental retardation, ectodermal dysplasia, poor dentition, congenital heart disease, polydactyly, and syndactyly are the major components of this syndrome. The condition is familial, and occurs more frequently in the Amish people of Pennsylvania.

Marfan's syndrome

Characterized by unusually long digits (arachnodactyly) and hypermobility of the joints. High arched palate, scolosis, and subluxation of ocular lenses are common. They have a high risk for thoracic aneurysms. The condition is phenotypically identical to homocystinuria.

Arthrogryposis multiplex congenita

Involves fibrous ankylosis of most of the joints of the body. Muscular development is poor. Usually have normal mentality, but activity can be severely restricted.

Osteogenesis imperfecta

In the severe fetal type (osteogenesis imperfecta congenita) fractures may occur in utero, and are common during birth. Growth retardation occurs because of recurrent fractures. Mentality is normal. Blue sclerae are characteristic findings. Inhereitance is usually autosomal dominant.

Foot problems

Posturing is the habitual position in which one holds the foot, however, it can be manipulated into normal position. A deformity is present if the foot cannot be manually manipulated into normal position.

Flatfoot (pes planus)

If a longitudinal arch is present when the child is not weight bearing, the arch will develop normally and no treatment is needed.

Cavovarus foot

An unusually high longitudinal arch of the foot. Neurologic abnormalities such as Charcot-Marie-Tooth disease, Friedreich's ataxia and diastematomyelia should be ruled out.

Pigeon toes

Toeing in of the foot may be due to posturing or deformity of the foot, tibia or the femur.

Metatarsus adductus

Positional deviation of the forefoot that can be corrected by manipulation. Serial casting may be needed to prevent development of a high arch with medial inclination of the heel.

Metatarsus varus

Medial deformity of the forefoot that cannot be corrected by manipulation, since it is due to an intrauterine subluxation of tarsometaatarsal joints with adduction and inversion of the metatarsal bones. Serial casting or surgery may are needed to prevent development of a high arch with medial inclination of the heel.

Talipes Equinovarus (clubfoot)

The foot is pointed downward (like a horse: equinus=horse), with medial deviation of the forefoot and medial inversion of the heel. Spontaneous correction does not occur. Aggressive treatment is indicated. Those not responding to serial casting will require surgical correction.

Talipes Calcaneovalgus

The reverse of club foot. This is a benign condition due to intrauterine molding pressures. The foot is everted and dorsiflexed at the ankle. Passive stretching usually results in correction. Casting is rarely indicated.

Lower leg problems

Tibial torsion

The tibia is normally internally rotated and bowed until about 9 years of age.

Blount Disease

A disturbance of the growth plate at the proximal tibia. More common in those with precocious walking and African ancestry. If not corrected with braces and/or surgery, it can leave permanent deformities.

Osgood-Schlatter's disease

Tenderness and swelling over the tibial tuberosity due to fibrocartilage microfractures at the insertion of the patellar tendon. It occurs in late childhood and early adolsecence, and is more common in males. The condition is generally benign, but pain may persist with activity for up to a year after skeletal maturity.

Knee problems

Osteochondritis dessicans

This is the result of necrosis and separation of bone adjacent to articular cartilage. The knee is a common site for it to occur, though it can also be found in talus, femoral head or lateral humeral condyle. The area is at risk for fractures.

Genu varum (bowleg)

Normal until about 2 years of age.

Genu valgum (knock knee)

Normal from 2 years until about 8 years of age.

Baker's cyst

Common popliteal cyst during middle childhood. Almost always benign.

Thigh problems

Femoral anteversion

A usual cause of toeing in after age 2 to 3 years. It refers to excessive internal rotation of the femur compared to external rotation. If there is no external rotation of the hip with it in extension, orthopedic evaluation is needed.

Leg length discrepancies

Shortening of a femur is a common cause of discrepancies in leg length. Orthopedic evaulation is indicated if the difference in leg lengths is greater than 2.5 cm.

Hip problems

Congenital dysplasia of the hip

Whether the hip is dislocatable or dislocated, it needs to be detected and treated before the child walks or permenant deformity will ensue.In the newborn period the Barlow test (a click is felt as the hip is adducted toward midline in a flexed position) is diagnostic. The Ortolani test (The hip is abducted away from midline, producing a click if the femoral head slips out of the acetabulum) is the opposite of the Barlow test and is confirmatory. Asymmetric gluteal folds and apparent shortening of the affected leg are also clues to the presence of this condition. More common in girls.

Slipped capital femoral epiphysis

A fracture through the physis of the femoral head can occur during the pubescent growth spurt. Shortening of the thigh and loss of internal rotation of the hip are characteristic findings of this condition. The volunerable age group is: males 10- 17 years; females 8-15 years. This condition is associated with the black race, males, obesity and hypothyriodism.

Legg-Perthes-Calve disease

Avascular necrosis of the femoral head. Persistent pain is common. The highest incidence is between 4 and 8 years of age during the period of rapid growth of the epiphysis. The incidence is 6 times greater in males than females.

Toxic synovitis

Transient synovitis is the most common cause of limp and hip in boys in the 3 to 10 year age range. It often follows an URI and has a normal erythrocyte sedimentation rate and normal WBC. Because symptoms, age, sex and laboratory are similar to that found in avascular necrosis of the hip and cannot be distinguished always from septic arthritis, serial hip x-rays or technetium bone scans and possibily joint aspiration are warranted.

Spine problems

Scolosis

Adolescent idiopathic scolosis has its onset after 10 years of age and can progress rapidly during the pubescent growth spurt. Females are at higher risk for progressive deformity. A history of pain should initiate search for lesions of the spinal cord or neoplasms, since the idiopathic condition is generally painless. Cases with curves more than 20 degrees should have orthopedic evaluation.

Torticollis

This condition is common in the neonatal period and is associated with a contracture of the sternocleidomastoid muscle. Torticollis may also be seen from gastroesopheal reflux (Sandifer syndrome) and with subluxations of cervical spine facettes. Hint: muscle spasm occurs on the side of shortening of the sternocleidomastoid in spastic torticollis and the opposite side in subluxation.

Klippel-Feil anomaly

The result of segmentation failure in the cervical spine. It has a high association with other anomalies, including cardiac lesions, urinary tract problems and auditory apparatus anomalies.

Diastematomyelia

The spinal cord is split and anchored in the spinal canal by bony or fibrous spicules. The result can be dysfunction of the bladder or lower extremity muscles. A hairy patch is often present over the affected area of the spine. A tethered spinal cord can produce similar problems.

Down syndrome subluxation of C1

Ligamentous laxity can occur in children with Down syndrome and place them at risk for subluxation of C1 on C2.

Elbow problems

Subluxation of the radial head

Referred to as nursemaid's elbow, this condition can occur when the toddler is picked up by the wrist. Then the child typically holds the arm by its side with the palm down (pronated) and refuses to use it until it is reduced by supination of the palm while flexing the elbow.

Elbow fractures

Supracohdylar fractures of the elbow are at high risk for development of the compartment syndrome (Volkman's contracture) if not adequately treated.

APPROACH TO PEDIATRIC EMERGENCIES

Thomas A. Lera

Initial Approach

Management of a critically ill or injured child demands a systematic approach. This systematic approach must include a plan to identify and begin emergent treatment for stabilization of the patient even before a complete history and physical examination are obtainable. In addition, a timely, directed evaluation of each body area must be performed in order to minimize the chance of overlooking potentially serious additional/contributing illnesses or injuries.

The above is accomplished utilizing a PRIMARY and SECONDARY SURVEY system. The PRIMARY SURVEY is an initial assessment of the status of the patient's airway, oxygenation, ventilation, circulation and neurologic status. During this phase, life-threatening problems are identified and because it is not uncommon to encounter serious physiologic alterations in the course of the primary Survey, it is frequently necessary to interrupt the order of the survey to perform resuscitative measures. In contrast, the SECONDARY SURVEY includes a detailed, timely complete physical exam. It surveys each body area in a head-to-toe fashion. Included here are a directed history, a brief past medical history, indicated lab and/or radiographic studies which may lead to a specific diagnosis or a list of problems which may require further attention.

Mneumonics based on the ABC's can help guide one in the performance of both of these surveys.

PRIMARY SURVEY

A.   AIRWAY

The goals of airway management are:
1.   Recognition and relief of obstruction
2.   Promotion of adequate gas exchange
3.   Prevention of aspiration of gastric contents
4.   Attention to protection of the cervical spine

Treatment/Therapeutic modalities
   a) Triple Airway Maneuver: tilt head back, displace mandible forward open mouth (jaw thrust alone with suspected neck injuries - NOTE: the tongue is the most common obstruction to the pediatric airway)
   b)   Use oral suction cautiously; may need oro-pharyngeal airway
   c)   Endotracheal intubation; cricothyroidotomy

B.   BREATHING/VENTILATION

1.   Observe for adequate gas exchange - look, listen, feel. Deficient air exchange must be rapidly diagnosed and treated. The following mneumonic addresses treatable causes of inadequate breathing:

Cause	Intervention
A irway obstruction	jaw thrust
T ension pneumothorax	aspiration/chest tube
O pen pneumothorax	aspiration/chest tube
M assive pneumothorax	aspiration/chest tube
F lail chest	postitive pressure ventilation
C ardiac tamponade	pericardiocenters
G astric distension	NG tube

2.   Methods to augment ventilation:
   a)   Mouth to mask (over patients mouth/nose) breathing
   b)   Bag-valve-mask ventilation
   c)   Endotracheal intubation with mechanical ventilation
   d)   Cricothyrotomy (needle/surgical)

3.   Generous use of O_2 (100%) is warranted initially in almost all emergency settings NOTE: Children will electively place themselves in a position of maximal airway comfort when allowed/able to do so. Do not change this position unnecessarily until more definite airway/breathing measures are available.

4.   Oxygen should be supplied by a means that meets the patient's needs i.e., percent of O_2 needed <u>AND</u> that is acceptable to the patient eg: hood, nasal prongs, face mask, shield, cannula, etc.

C.   CIRCULATION

Major Goals
1.   Assess overall circulatory status - note the quality, rate and regularity of the pulses - centrally and peripherally. Determine capillary refill time and blood pressure (NOTE: blood pressure is an insensitive measure of adequate circulation in children until profound deficiencies exists -compromised circulation can and does exist despite a normal blood pressure.)

<u>Tx</u>:   Circulatory support: diagnose and control both external and internal hemorrhage:
   a)   Control active hemorrhage - direct pressure
   b)   IVF, crystalloid/colloid/blood
   c)   MAST suit application(s)
   d)   External cardiac massage (CPR)
   e)   Defibrillation

2.   Obtain reliable venous access: IV/IO access
         Blood for lab studies, including Type and Crossmatch

D.   DISABILITY (DE-BRAIN)

1.   Rapid screening of neurological system is essential. Obtain "neuro vital signs": assessment of pupillary response; level of consciousness [Alert, Verbal response, Pain response, Unresponsive]; notation of localized signs

2.   Calculation of Glasgow Coma Scale can be used

E.   EXPOSURE/ENVIRONMENT

1.   Complete physical exam requires complete removal of clothing. Children cool rapidly because of their large surface to body ratio. Maintain temperature by radiant warmer or warming blanket at 36-37°C.

2.   Address hypo-hyperthermia as needed

F.   FOLEY CATHETER
- do not place if blood at urinary meatus or with suspected pelvic fracture

G.   GASTRIC   DECOMPRESSION   -   OROGASTRIC/NASOGASTRIC TUBES
- do not place if suspected facial fractures present
- <u>always</u> confirm placement

H.   HISTORY

Obtain an **A M P L E** history
A llergies
M edication
P ast medical illness
L ast medication
E vents surrounding illness/injury

SECONDARY SURVEY

I.   DETAILED PHYSICAL EXAM

A.   HEAD (HEENT)

1. Maxillofacial trauma - palpate bony prominences; evidence for bloody or CSF discharge from nose, mouth, ears; nasal septal hematoma; check dentition; suspect basilar skull fracture with Battle's sign, racoon eyes, hemotympanum
2. Dehydration - sunken fontanelle and/or eyes
3. Eyes - pupillary size and reaction, visual acuity, fundal exam
4. Scalp - exam for lacerations/hematomas
5. Fontanelle - sunken: dehydration
   - bulging: may indicate increased ICP, meningitis/sepsis

B.   NECK

Palpate for obvious signs of fracture/dislocation and midline position of trachea; examine for SQ emphysema, hematoma, localized pain; assess for JVD; [NECK/C-SPINE FILMS]

C.   CHEST

1. Evaluate visually for adequacy of respiratory excursion, asymmetry of chest wall motion or presence of a flail segment
2. Carefully palpate chest wall and auscultate lung fields and heart
3. R/O Pulmonary/Myocardial contusion, Aortic/Tracheobronchial/Esophageal disruptions; [CHEST FILMS]
4. Examine/assess respiratory adequacy by: skin color, nasal flaring, use of accessary muscles, grunting, stridor, wheezing, positioning of child

D.   ABDOMEN

1. Initial exam: inspect for ease of abdominal wall movement with respiration, gentle palpation, auscultation of bowel sounds
2. Observe and palpate flanks
3. Serial examinations are often needed to establish a definitive diagnosis
4. Investigate pregnancy and its related problems with female patients

E.   PELVIS

1. Palpate bony prominences for tenderness, instability
2. Exam perineum for laceration, hematoma, acute bleeding or discharge
3. Check urethral meatus for blood
4. Child/sexual abuse

F.   RECTUM

Evaluate integrity of wall, prostatic injury, muscle tone, occult GI hemorrhage; child abuse

F. **EXTREMITIES**
1. Exam for signs of abrasion, contusion, hematoma, soft tissue injuries
2. Exam for bony instability and neurovascular function
3. Exam for fractures/dislocations

G. **BACK**
Exam with neck/spinal immobilization as indicated **NOTE:** this is accomplished if no obvious spinal cord injury or paralysis is present

H. **SKIN**
1. Exam for bruises/petechiae - color, size, "age" may be suggestive of trauma, coagulopathy, physical abuse
2. Rash - hemorrhagic, stellate, or rapidly expanding may indicate life-
threatening illnesses (eg: meningococcemia, septic shock, anaphylaxis, etc.)
3. Burns

I. **NEUROLOGIC**
1. In-depth neuro exam: motor, sensory, cranial nerve and level of consciousness determinations
2. Exam tympanic membranes, nose for basilar skull fracture
3. Fundi exam
4. Presence of spinal cord trauma

II. **DETAILED HISTORY** - as appropriate and available

III. **RADIOGRAPHIC & LAB STUDIES** - based on physical finding in $1^0/2^0$ survey and history; may need serial exams and more sophisticated studies eg: computed tomography

IV. **MONITORING** - continuous monitoring and frequent reevaluation are a must

V. **LIST FINDINGS** - documentation of initial assessments and resuscitation procedures; list additional areas needing consultation/investigate

VI. **DEFINITIVE CARE** - in hospital care; determine need for operative intervention and/or intensive care admission

EMERGENCY EVALUATION AND MANAGEMENT OF SELECTED ORGAN SYSTEM FAILURES

I.   **RESPIRATORY SYSTEM FAILURE: ACUTE RESPIRATORY FAILURE**

CRITERIA   RR >90/min (<12 mos)
RR >70/min ($\geq$12 mos)
P_aO_2 <40 torr (in absence of cyanotic heart disease)
PCO_2 >65 torr
Mechanical Ventilation
Tracheal Intubation

DEFINITION   clinical condition marked by inadequate O_2 elimination and/or inadequate oxygenation of blood

ETIOLOGIC CLASSIFICATION

1. LUNG FAILURE: diseases affecting airways, alveoli, capillary membranes, pulmonary circulation
2. RESPIRATORY PUMP FAILURE: disease along the pathway from brain stem to respiratory center to spinal cord, phrenic nerves to chest wall muscles

---

Common Causes of Respiratory Failure in Children

Lung Failure:

o Upper airway obstruction

o Bronchiolitis

o Asthma

o Pneumonia

o Bronchopulmonary dysplasia

o Adult Respiratory Distress Syndrome

Pump Failure:

o Drug Overdose

o CNS Disease

o Neuromuscular Disorders

EVALUATION - physical exam is most important tool
- pulse oximetry (continuous/intermittent) gives information regarding oxygen saturation (O_2 sat <90 = PO_2 <60)
- lab tests may include arterial blood gases; CXR

Typical Physical Exam and Arterial Blood Gas in Acute Respiratory Failure

Signs & Symptoms	Blood Gas
o Tachypnea/Dyspnea	o PO_2 <60 mmHg (FIO_2 0.6)
o Intercostal Retractions	o PCO_2 >45 mmHg
o Diminished Breath Sounds	o pH <7.3
o Cyanosis	
o Altered sensorium	

EXAMPLES OF EMERGENT PROBLEMS
1. Asthma (Hyperreactive Airways Disease)
2. BPD (Bronchopulmonary Dysplasia)
3. Bronchiolitis especially Respiratory Syncytial Virus
4. ARDS (Adult Respiratory Distress Syndrome)
5. Upper Airway Obstruction: CNS dysfunction; anatomic causes; infectious (croup, epiglottis); trauma; foreign body aspiration; burns; anaphylaxis/laryngospasm

MANAGEMENT

Guidelines for Initiating Mechanical Ventilation
1. Ventilator type: volume or pressure controlled
   NOTE: generally the type of ventilator and kind of support depend upon patient characteristics eg: age, weight, reason for need for support, pathophysiology of disease process, time/point in disease process

2. Initial Ventilator Settings:
   A. No Pulmonary Disease:
   1. Pressure Ventilator
      a. Peak Pressure .... 16 - 24
      b. PEEP .... 0 - 5
      c. Rate .... Age Dependent
      d. I:E Ratio .... 1:1-1:2 (Never > 1 sec)
      e. FiO_2 .... ≤0.30

   2. Volume Ventilator
      a. Tidal Volume .... 8 - 15ml/kg
      b. PEEP .... 0 - 5
      c. Rate .... Age Dependent
      d. Insp Time (%) .... 25 - 33
      e. FiO_2 .... ≤0.30

B. With Pulmonary Disease:
  1. Begin with ventilator set at above settings except
     $FiO_2 = 1.0$
  2. Adjust based upon
     a. Physical examination
     b. Non-invasive monitors Oximetry/capnography
     c. Arterial blood gases (Capillary blood gases)

ENDOTRACHEAL INTUBATION
M-S-M-A-I-D

All equipment at bedside and functioning

MASK	**Appropriate size with bag and O_2**
SUCTION	**Tonsillar tip and Tracheal**
MACHINE	**Appropriate for patient's size and problem**
AIRWAY	**Laryngscope, Blade & ET Tubes** **Tube Size = 16 + Age in years/4** **Tape, Benzoin** **< 8 years old, use uncuffed tube**
IV	**Patient and Secure**
DRUGS	**For Intubation and Resuscitation**

**ALWAYS CHECK & RE-CHECK BREATH SOUNDS
FOLLOWING INTUBATION**

CARDIOVASCULAR SYSTEM FAILURE: SHOCK

CRITERIA
MAP <40mmHg (<12 mos)
MAP <50mmHg ≥12 mos
HR <50BPM <12 mos
HR <40BPM ≥12 mos
Cardiac arrest
Need for continued vasoactive drug infusion

DEFINITION
Syndrome of acute homeostatic derangement of various etiologies involving multiple organ systems, which ultimately causes failure of cellular metabolism **NOTE:** shock is <u>not</u> <u>necessarily</u> decreased intravascular volume

ETIOLOGY - CLASSIFICATION

1. Hypovolemia
    a. Vomiting/diarrhea
    b. Hemorrhagic
2. Cardiogenic
3. Neurogenic
4. Septic

DIFFERENTIAL DIAGNOSIS OF THE SEPTIC-APPEARING INFANT

Infections
Meningitis
Bacterial sepsis
Viral infection
Urinary tract infection

Cardiac
Dysrhythmias
Supraventricular tachycardia
Atrioventricular block
Congenital heart disease
Pulmonary hypertension
Cardiomyopathies
Myocarditis
Infiltrative disease

Metabolic
Electrolyte disturbances
Hypoglycemia/Hyperglycemia
Inborn errors of metabolism

Gastrointestinal
Intestinal obstruction or ischemia
Gastroenteritis with dehydration
Vomiting

Miscellaneous
Child abuse, shaken child syndrome
Anemia
Hepatic failure, Reye's syndrome
Intracranial bleed

	Classification of Severity of Shock in Children			
	I	**II**	**III**	**IV**
Estimated blood volume deficit	10-15%	15-30%	30-40%	>40%
Pulse (bpm)	>100	>120	>150	>150
Resp	normal	increased	marked increase	tachypneic/ apneic
Capillary refill (sec)	<4	> 4	> 6 - 8	> 10
Blood pressure	normal	narrowed pulse pressure	hypotensive	severely hypotensive to absent
Mentation	normal	anxious	confused	unconscious
Orthostatic hypotension	+	++	+++	++++
Urine output (ml/kg)	1-3	0.5-1	<0.5	none

EVALUATION

```
+------------------------------------------------------+
|                                                      |
|            Signs and Symptoms of Shock               |
|                                                      |
|      Vasoconstriction          Pallor                |
|      Acrocyanosis              Sweating              |
|      Poor peripheral pulses    Ileus                 |
|      Altered consciousness     Oliguria              |
|                                                      |
+------------------------------------------------------+
```

SPECIFIC TYPES

1. Hypovolemic Shock
    - most common cause of shock in children
    - blood pressure is an <u>insensitive</u> index of hypovolemic
    - treatment plan:

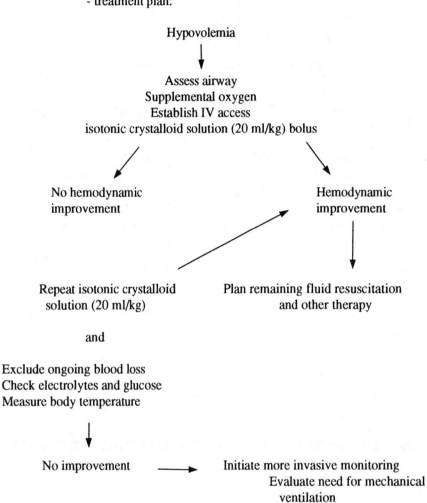

Hypovolemia

Assess airway
Supplemental oxygen
Establish IV access
isotonic crystalloid solution (20 ml/kg) bolus

No hemodynamic
improvement

Hemodynamic
improvement

Repeat isotonic crystalloid
solution (20 ml/kg)

Plan remaining fluid resuscitation
and other therapy

and

Exclude ongoing blood loss
Check electrolytes and glucose
Measure body temperature

No improvement

Initiate more invasive monitoring
Evaluate need for mechanical
ventilation

- hemorrhagic type - internal blood loss -
  consider
  intracranial/intra abdominal/intrathoresis/retroperitoneal causes
- volume loss type - acute gastroenteritis (Vomiting/Diarrhea) most
  common

2. Cardiogenic Shock
- acute hypoperfusion and acidosis caused by heart failure which occurs when cardiac chambers are not adequately filled in a normovolemic child or if the ventricles cannot eject a sufficient proportion of their volume; failure of both filling and ejection can have traumatic and non-traumatic etiologies
- management: Vasopressors   eg: Dopamine, Dobutamine, Epinephrine, Amrinone

    Fluids
    Arrhythmia/Dysrhythmia Management

3. Neurogenic Shock
- warm extremeties; slow pulse relative to low blood pressure
- hypotension due to diminished or absent SNS activity and loss of vascular tone
- classic example is shock following transection of spinal cord
- management: Trendelenberg position
    Fluids
    Vasopressors   eg: Phenylephrine, Ephedrine

4. Septic Shock
- shock from overwhelming bacteremia and/or septicemia
- most commonly associated with Gram-negative organisms - but may be seen with Gram-positive infections as well as fulminant viral infections

Bacteremia and endotoxemia characteristically progress through two phases of shock: a "warm" phase and a "cold" phase. Their effect on the vascular and cellular permeability is to initially produce capillary leak and systemic vasodilitation. This is clinically manifest as a "warm" phase of shock; the extremeties are flushed and warm but there is a decreased preload to the heart. If this condition persists, the decreased cardiac output leads to hypoperfusion which in turn leads to tissue anaerobic metabolism, metabolic acidosis and release of myocardial depressant factors. The resulting vasoconstriction is seen clinically as the "cold" phase of septic shock.

===
Clinical Clues for Sepsis
===

o Clinical suspicion or evidence for infection
o Temperature instability (fever or hypothermia)
o Tachycardia/Tachypnea
o Impaired organ system function
    peripheral hypoperfusion   hypoxemia
    altered level of consciousness   acidosis
    oliguria
                          pulmonary edema
- management: Fluids
    Vasopressors   eg: Dopamine, Dobutamine, Epinephrine
    Antibiotic/Antiviral therapy

Clinical Differentiation of types shock		
	Skin appearance	**Cervical veins**
Hypovolemic	Pale, cold, clammy	Flat
Cardiogenic	Pale, cold, clammy	Bulging
Neurogencic	Pink, Warm, dry	Normal
Septic	Flushed, warm, dry then,cold, clammy	Variable

CONGESTIVE HEART FAILURE

DEFINITION   Inability of heart to pump adequate blood volume for the circulatory and metabolic needs of the body

ETIOLOGY   Commonly it results from:
Volume overload - increased preload or excessive intravascular volume
Pressure overload - increased afterload or increased vascular resistance
Myocardial dysfunction - 2^0 congenital lesions or acqusic cardiomyopathy or myocarditis
Dysrhythmias

- 90% of children who develop congestive heart failure do so in the 1st year of life as a result of congenital heart disease

- other etiologies include: cor pulmonale from chronic lung disease (eg: bronchopulmonary dysplasia), cardiomyopathy, electrolyte abnormalities, endocarditis or rheumatic carditis, renal failure, systemic hypertension, anemia, hyperthyroidism, and overhydration.

EVALUATION Assessment: decreased exercise tolerance, altered behavior, weight loss, change in eating habits
Exam: tachycarida, +/- gallop rhythm, cardiomegaly, venous congestion (hepatomegaly, JVD, edema) tachypnea with rales, rhonchi, wheezing, orthopnea, exercise intolerance
Diagnosis: chest X-ray, electrocardiography, arterial blood gas, echocardiography

MANAGEMENT Improve contractility while reducing afterload.
1. Inotropic Agents: Digitalis
Fluids
Dopamine/Dobutamine
2. Reduction of Preload (Volume Overload): fluid restriction
diuretic therapy
3. Reduction of Afterload (Pressure Overload):
- sodium nitroprusside

Basic CPR in Infants and Children
(for children > 8 years: AHA recommends CPR be performed as on would in an adult)

Infant (< 1 year)	**Older Child** (1-8 years)

Airway

Determine unresponsiveness
Call for help
Position patient supine.
Support head and neck.
Head-tilt/chin lift or Jaw thrust.
No blind finger sweeps.

Breathing

2 initial breaths

Then: **20 breaths/min**	Then: **15 breaths/min**

Circulation

Check **brachial**/femoral pulse	Check **carotid**/femoral pulse

Activate EMS System

Compression location: **1 finger breadth below** **intermammary line on sternum**	Compression location: **lower 1/3 of sternum**
Compression method: **2 fingers on sternum or** **hands encircle sternum**	Compression method: **1 or 2 hands on sternum**
Compression depth: **0.5-1"**	Compression depth: **1-1.5"**
Compression rate: **100/min**	Compression rate: **80-100/min**

Compression: ventilation ratio = 5:1
Reassessment: Palpate pulse every 10 cycles

NEUROLOGIC SYSTEM FAILURE: CENTRAL NERVOUS SYSTEM FAILURE

CRITERIA	Glasgow Coma Scale < 5
	Fixed, Dilated pupils
	ICP > 20 torr (for > 20 min)

CLASSIFICATION/DEFINITIONS

Stupor: state of unresponsiveness - patient can be aroused by vigorous stimulation

Coma: state of unresponsiveness - patient <u>cannot</u> be aroused

Assessment of Altered State of Consciousness: more informative to indicate specific stimuli required for response (**A**lert, **V**oice, **P**ain, Unresponsive)

Common causes of Coma in Infants and Children

Pneumonic: TIPS on the Vowels

A -- **Alcohol:** Not only the aldolscent patient is at risk for depressed levels of consciousness from alcohol. Infants may adsorb enough alcohol through the skin from alcohol baths or from alcohol containing medications to cause coma.

E -- **Epilepsy (and other causes of seizures):** Both postictal states and continued subtle seizure activity without overt motor manifestations can cause the appearance of coma in the infant and child.

I -- **Insulin (hypo- or hyperglycemia):** Infants without adequate hepatic glycogen stores or depressed gluconeogenesis may sucumb to hypoglycemia as the result of various disease processes. Hyperglycemia can also cause coma. A fingerstick glucose is indicated in all comatose children.

I -- **Intussusception:** A vacant blank stare is often seen in the child with intussusception.

O -- **Overdose:** Drug overdose may be intentional, accidental or the result of misguided attempts at recreational use. They can even be acquried transplacentally at birth. A toxic drug screen is indicated in all cases of coma without clear etiology.

U -- **Uremia (and other metabolic causes):** A serum ammonia and electrolytes are often helpful in providing clues to metabolic causes of coma.

T -- **Trauma:** In comatose infants, retinal hemorrhages should alert the examiner to the possibility of intracranial trauma due to a "shaken baby" or other form of abuse. Intracranial bleeds or cerebral edema resulting from trauma that caused hypoxia or shock may be assessed by a CT of the head.

I -- **Infection:** Infection is more common as a cause of altered sensorium in children than adults. A high index of suspicion should lead to a lumbar puncture as soon as the probalility of increased intracranial pressure is excluded.

P -- **Psychiatric:** Factitious altered sensorium is exceedingly rare in children. It should be diagnosed by positive supporting evidence, not by lack of any other explanation for the an altered level of consciousness.

S -- **Stroke, shock, and other cardiovascular causes:** An altered level of consciousness can be caused by shock resulting in inadequate brain perfusion or by local cerebrovasular accidents. Hypertensive encephalopathy can cause a stroke like picture.

- Stupor, Coma and Altered States of Consciousness are signs of "brain failure," they should be treated emergently in an effort to minimize irrversable CNS injury.

MANAGEMENT Goals:
1. Prevent secondary hypoxic-ischemic brain injury
2. Prevent herniation
3. Diagnosis and treatment (if possible) underlying cause of coma

CEREBRAL PROTECTION/RESUSCITATION

Ensure Airway, Breathing

Treat Hypotension
(Shock causes cerebral edema, cerebral edema does not cause shock)

a. colloid

b. dobutamine (10 mcg/kg/min)

Check Glasgow Coma Scale (GCS) and CNS Vital Signs (Record)

R/O Mass Lesion (CT Scan When Stable)

Treat Hyperthermia

GCS $\leq$ 7
Consider Invasive ICP Monitoring
and
Cerebral Protection Resuscitation

GCS $\geq$ 8
Observe <u>Closely</u> Clinically
Breathing Patterns
Pupils
E.O.M.
Posturing
Re-Calculate GSC

Attempt to Keep CPP (MAP - ICP) > 60

Factors important in ICP Reduction:

1. Hyperventilate (pCO_2 25-30)
2. Elevate HOB 30 degrees
3. Sedation and/or paralysis
4. Lidocaine for attenuation of ICP (1.5-3 mg/kg)
5. Mannitol (0.5 - 1.0 gm/kg IV)
6. Lasix (1 - 2 mg/kg IV)
7. Barbiturate (sedative dose Nembutal 2 mg/kg)
8. Hypothermia (core temp 33 degrees C)

===
Indications for Intubation of the Comatose Child
===

      o Inability to maintain patent airway

      o Glasgow Coma Scale < 8

      o Absent cough reflex

      o Absent gag reflex

      o Hypoxemia with adequate supplemental oxygen

      o Hypoventilation

      o Impending brainstem herniation (hyperventilation Rx)

===

DIAGNOSIS:

Glasgow Coma Scale

Response	Adults & Children	Infants	Points
Eye Opening	no response	no response	1
	to pain	to pain	2
	to voice	to voice	3
	spontaneous	spontaneous	4
Verbal	no response	no response	1
	incomprehensible	moans to pain	2
	inappropriate words	cries to pain	3
	disoriented conversation	irritable	4
	oriented and appropriate	coos, babbles	5
Motor	no response	no response	1
	decerebrate posturing	decerebrate posturing	2
	decorticate posturing	decorticate posturing	3
	withdraws to pain	withdraws to pain	4
	localizes pain	withdraws to touch	5
	obeys commands	normal spontaneous movements	6
Total Score			3-15

SPINAL CORD TRAUMA
    Pediatric spinal cord injuries are unusual. They are most commonly seen with MVA

(motor vehicle accidents) in < 10 year old age group; in those > 10 years - MVAs as well as recreational and organized sporting accidents account for the majority of spinal cord injuries

The neurological evaluation for suspected spinal cord injury includes:

1. **History**
   A spinal injury should be assumed until proved otherwise in any comatose child. Children who are awake and complaining of neck or back pain or radicular pain, dysesthesias or numbness also are possible candidates to for a spinal injury.

2. **Examination**
   a. Palpate for tenderness of the neck or spine in awake older children.
   b. A careful evaluation of the movement of the extremities, sensation, and reflexes in awake children should be done.

3. Any child who is awake and flaccid has a spinal cord injury until proven otherwise.

4. Hypotension can result from loss of vasomotor tone due to a cervical cord injury.

Management objectives are to prevent injury or further injury to the spinal cord and to address the present neural injury. This is accomplished in general by:

1. **Immobilization**
   The cervical spine should be immobilized as soon as feasible at the scene. It should remain immobilized during resuscitation efforts and radiographic evaluation until these studies and thorough neurologic evaluation indicate that it is safe to remove this restraint. An adequate C-spine x-ray requires visualization of all 7 cervical vertebrae.

2. **Airway**
   The airway should be protected and intubation must be done without moving the neck. If no facial injuries are present nasotracheal intubation may be the method of choice. Rarely, a cricothyroidltomy may be the only option.

3. **Blood Pressure**
   Blood pressure should be monitored and supported. Children who are hypotensive from a spinal cord injury should be treated with vasopressors and not volume resuscitation.

4. **Other Considerations**
   Gastric dilatation is seen with cervical and thoracic cord injury, and may compromise ventilation if not relieved. Distension of the urinary bladder occurs with lower spinal cord injury and catheterization may be necessary.

   NOTE: The early use of relatively high-dose steroids is advocated for some spinal cord injuries. Prompt neurosurgical intervention should be obtained when these patients are encountered.

HEMATOLOGIC SYSTEM FAILURE (HEMATOPOIETIC)

CRITERIA Hgb < 5 g/dl

WBC < 3000 cells/mm^3

Platelets < 20,000/mm^3

DIC (PT > 20 sec/PTT > 60 sec)

Fluid Replacement in Hematologic Shock:

Initially replace the volume loss with a balanced salt solution (RL, NS).
Give 10-20 ml/kg as a bolus, replacing 3 ml of crystalloid for every 1 ml of
circulatory blood volume lost.

The rationale for the "3 for 1" rule is that only approximately 1/3 of the infused
crystalloid remains in the intravascular space - SIMILARLY-when one is going
to give packed Red Blood Cells (PRBCs) they are usually given in 10 ml/kg
transfusions for each three doses of crystalloid at 20 ml/kg. Last blood volume
can also be replaced on a ml for ml basis with whole blood (preferred when
available).

RENAL FAILURE: ACUTE RENAL FAILURE (AFR)

CRITERIA BUN > 100 mg/dl

Serum Creatinine > 2 mg/dl

Dialysis

Diagnosis and Management of Acute Renal Failure is covered in the Chapter on
RENAL DISORDERS

I.   HYPERTENSIVE CRISIS

Hypertension in children is rare but should not be missed. It is defined as Systolic, diastolic or mean arterial pressures that fall above the upper limit of normal (> 95%) for the patients age. Careful attention must be given to the proper technique used to obtain blood pressure - especially in infants and small children.

Classification of hypertensive crisis

> Hypertensive Emergency
> > This condition has life threatening end organ (CNS, cardiac, renal)
> > > involvement and needs to be corrected within minutes to hours.
> > Hypertensive encephalopathy
> > Malignant hypertension
> > Acute complications of accelerated hypertension
> > > pulmonary edema
> > > Cerebrovascular accident with hemorrhage or infarction
> > Eclampsia
> > Pheochromocytoma
> Hypertensive Urgency
> > No evidence of life threatening end organ involvement; needs to be
> > > corrected in hours to days.
> > > Renal failure or impairment
> > > Acute glomerulonephritis
> > > Preeclampsia
> > > Postoperative bleeding
> > > Newly developed hypertension

For the child over 2 years of age:

Hypertension is present if the Diastolic Pressure is   >   (80 + age in years)

ASSESSMENT

1.   Do not use too small a blood pressure cuff. The width of bladder on the blood pressure cuff should be at least 2/3 the length of the upper arm.

2.   Obtain a history to uncover possible underling etiology of the hypertension (eg: renal disease, coarctation, pheochromocytoma, Cushing's disease, drug effect, neurofibromatosis).

3.   Physical exam should include four-extremity blood pressures, evaluation for

end organ injury such as fundoscopic changes, decreased visual acuity, congestive heart failure, abdominal bruit, motor or sensor disturbances, and potential causes such as cafe au lait spots.

4. Obtain urinalysis, electrolyte,s BUN, creatinine, chest x-ray, EKG and if CNS involvement, a CT of the head.. If the patients condition permits consider obtaining renin level prior to beginning antihypertensive therapy.

5. Patients with blood pressure >95th percentile require further evaluation and may require therapy. Patients with evidence of target organ injury (eg: headache, vomiting, epistaxis, decreased visual acuity, fundoscopic changes, congestive heart failure, proteinuria) or blood pressure significantly >95th percentile require immediate monitoring and treatment.

   NOTE: In patients being evaluated for Hypertensive Cerebrovascular Syndromes: when a patient presents with hypertension and an alteration in mental status - the hypertension work-up and emergent control should take precedent over the work-up for the change in mental status. Entities associated with HTCVS include: hypertensive encephalopathy, intracerebral hemorrhage, subarchnoid hemorrhage, head/neck trauma, side effects from recreational durgs and neoplasms.

6. If possible, secure IV access before beginning therapy. (Niphedipine can be given sublingually to vomiting patients).

COMMON HYPERTENSION CAUSES BY AGE

Neonate:	coarctation of aorta renovascular disease intracranial hemorrhage
Infants ≤ 2 yrs:	renovascular disease intrinsic renal disease coarctation of aorta neuroblastoma
2-8 yrs:	renovascular disease intrinsic renal diagnosis
> 8 yrs:	renovascular disease intrinsic renal disease essential hypertension

TREATMENTS

1.   Blood pressure should not be decreased by greater than one third of the total goal over the first 4-6h.

2.   Patients with underlying chronic hypertension may have a shifted autoregulatory curve and require increased blood pressures to maintain normal cerebral perfusion. Therefore, elevated pressure should be lowered more slowly in these patients.

3.   Drugs

Drug	Dose	Comments
Diazoxide arteriolar vasodilator	1-3 mg/kg rapid IVP (undiluted) q 15-20 min x 2-3 doses	First line drug. May be given in ER setting NOTE: give with furosemide to avoid rebound hypertension.
Labetalol alpha and beta blocker	1-3 mgkghr IV	First line drug. May require ICU setting
Nitroprusside arteriolar and venous vasodilator	0.5-8.0 mcg/kg/min IV	Very short half-life Allows tight control of BP reduction. Requires ICU monitoring.
Hydralazine arteriolar vasodilator	0.1-0.2 mg/kg IV	Second line drug. Maintains cerebral, renal, coronary, and uterine perfusion.
Phentolamine alpha blocker	0.1-0.2 mg/kg IV Increase dose as needed Effective dose may vary among patients	Use in suspected excess catecholeamine states.
Nifedipine Ca^{++} channel blocker	0.25-0.5 mg/kg SL	Can be given SL in vomiting patients.
Minoxidil arteriolar vasodilator	2.5-5.0 mg PO	Consider in refractory renovascular hypertension

II.   HYPERKALEMIA

ETIOLOGY

Increased Stores		Normal Stores
Increased Urine K	**Decreased Urine K**	
Cell breakdown	Renal Failure	Leukocytosis
Transfusion with	Hypoaldosteronism	Thrombocytosis >750K/mm^3
aged blood	Aldosterone	Metabolic acidosis
NaCl substitutes	insensitivity	Cell lysis from blood drawing
	Decreased insulin	
	K-sparing diuretics	

SYMPTOMS

Serum K$^+$	ECG Changes	Other Symptoms
2.5	AV conduction defect, prominent U wave, ventricular arrhythmia, S-T segment depression	Apathy, weakness, parethesias
~7.5	T-wave elevation	greater weakness, paresthesias
~8	Loss of P wave, widening of QRS	
~9	S-T depression, further widening of QRS	Tetany, carpalspasm
~10	Bradycardia, sine-wave QRS-T, 1^0 AV block, ventricular arrhythmia, cardiac arrest	

ASSESSMENT

1.   Symptoms: Weakness, paresthesias, tetany.

2.   Progression of ECG changes: T-wave elevation, loss of P wave, widening QRS, S-T depression, further widened QRS, bradycardia, sine-wave QRS-T, 1st degree AV Block, ventricular arrhythmia, cardiac arrest.

TREATMENT

Drug	Dose and route	Onset (duration)	Mode of action	Comment
Calcuim Gluconate 10% (100mg/ml)	20 mg/kg IV over 5 minutes may repeat x 2	Immediate (30-60 min)	Stabilizes Cell Membranes	CaCl can worsen acidosis Monitor for bradycardia Hold infusion if heart rate drops < 100.
Sodium Bicarbonate 7.5% (1mEq/cc)	1-2 mEq/kg IV	20 min (1-4 hours)	Enhances intracellular transport of K	Assure adequate ventilation Will precipate if given with Calcium.
Glucose + Insulin	1-2 g/kg (5-10cc/kg 20% dextrose) 0.3 units/g glucose Adminster by infusion together over 2 hours	15-30 min (3-6 hours)	Enhances intraclualar transport of K	Monitor blood glucose
Sodium polystyrene sulfonate (Kayexalate)	1g/kg P.O. in 70% sorbitol or P.R. in 30% sorbitol every 6 hours		Exchanges K for Na in the intestine	Monitor for soduim overload
Dialysis		Time required for vascular access	Removes K from serum	Can also correct metabolic acidosis and fluid overload problems

GASTROINTESTINAL SYSTEM FAILURE

I.   HEPATIC FAILURE: ACUTE LIVER FAILURE

CRITERIA

Total Bili > 5 mg/dl and
SGOT or LDH more than 2 x normal
Hepatic encephalopathy ≥ grade II

CLASSIFICATION

==

ACUTE HEPATIC FAILURE - HEPATIC ENCEPHALOPATHY GRADING

==

Grade	Description	Mentation	Tremor/ Asterixis	EEG
I	Prodrome	Euphoria, occasional depression, confusion; slow mentation, offset; disordered speech; sleep pattern reversal	Slight	Normal
II	Impending coma	Stage I signs amplified; sleepy; inappropriate behavior, combative; loss of sphincter control	Present (easily elicited)	Generalized slowing
III	Stupor	Rousable, but generally asleep; incoherent speech; marked confusion	Present (if patient cooperates)	Abnormal
IV	Coma	Responds to pain only or no response	Absent (usually)	Grossly Abnormal

==

TREATMENT

1. IV glucose for hypoglycemia
2. Fluid and electrolyte balance
3. Correction of coagulation defects - vitamin K
4. Treatment of hepatic encephalopathy - protein restriction, purge gastrointestinal tract, treat cerebral edema
5. Treat/prevent GI bleeding - NG tube, antacids, cimetidine
6. Treat/prevent sepsis - antibiotic coverage
7. Support respiratory failure
8. Avoid diuretics
9. Maintain adequate cardiovascular status
10. Maintain nutrition

II. GI HEMORRHAGE

Blood loss In excess of 20cc/kg in 24 hours, or the equivalent need in blood/fluid replacement, constitutes GI failure and demands prompt diagnosis and treatment interactions.

III. REYE'S SYNDROME

An acute and frequently fatal encephalopathy associated with abnormal line function tests and with the infiltration of fat = the liver, kidneys and other organs.

CLINICAL PICTURE

1. Prodromal illness appears.
2. Recurrent, protracted vomiting occurs.
3. Mental confusion and lethargy occurs.
4. Physical examination shows
   a) Hyperpnea
   b) No jaundice
   c) Dilated pupils that react sluggishly to light.
   d) Hepatomegaly
   e) yperreflexia
   f) Positive Babinski sign
   g) Alternation between decorticate and decerebrate posturing

5. Stages of coma

==

Staging of Encephalopathy of Reye's Syndrome

==

Stage	Mental Status	Response to Pain	Other CNS Findings
0	Biochemical dysfunction without clinical manifestations. Liver biopsy is abnormal.		
I	lethargic, follows verbal commands	Purposeful	Normal
II	Stuporous, combative, disoriented, delirious	Purposeful	Hyperventilates, hyperreflexic, dilated pupils
III	Obtunded, comatose	Decorticate	Pupils dilated and react to light, hypoventilation, normal to sluggish mentation
IV	Comatose	Decerebrate	Loss of oculocephalic reflex, dilated pupils with or without, extreme hypoventilation respiratory arrest, caloric reflex disconjugate, no corneal reflex.
V	Comatose	Unresponsive	Flaccid with or without seizures loss of brain stem reflex, Cheyne-Stokes respirations - apnea

==

6.   Laboratory findings show the following:
   a)   Moderately or markedly elevated SGOT, SGPT, and LDH levels
   b)   Moderately to markedly prolonged prothrombin time
   c)   Mildly to markedly elevated blood-ammonia level
   d)   Normal or minimally elevated serum total bilirubin (less than 3 mg/100 ml)
   e)   Mixed metabolic acidosis, respiratory alkalosis
   g)   Normal to mildly decreased hemoglobin, hematocrit, with an elevated white blood-cell count.
   h)   Cerebrospinal fluid appearing accellular, possible with low glucose level
   i)   EEG with diffuse, slow, high-voltage pattern

BASIC PRINCIPLES

1.   The patient with Reye's syndrome will often appear to be recovering from an antecedent illness when protracted vomiting occurs. Within the next 24 to 36 hours, central-nervous-system dysfunction appears and may rapidly progress.

2.   The defect in Reye's syndrome is not known. Viral agents have been implicated in many cases (eg: varicella, influenze B, Coxsackie viruses A and B, adenovirus 3, echo-viruses 2, 8, 11). Attention has also focused on endogenous toxins (eg: ammonia and free fatty acids), exogenous toxins (eg: aflatoxins), aspirin, and specific hereditary or acquired urea-cycle enzyme deficiency states (eg: decreased or absent activity of carbamyl phosphate synthetase and/or ornithine transcarbamylase). The incidence of Reye's has decreased markedly since use of aspirin has been curtailed in children.

3.   Mortality varies from 25% to 50%. If Stage IV coma is reached, survival rate is low. Of the survivors, fewer than 30% will have central-nervous-system sequelae, such as mental retardation and seizures. Infants have the highest mortality and complication rates.

4.   All patients require admission to an ICU capable of intracranial monitoring. Appropriate consultations must be rapidly obtainable.

MUSCULOSKELETAL SYSTEM FAILURE

I. DIFFERENCES IN THE CHILD'S SKELETON

A. Fracture Patterns
Cortex of the child's bone is porous and less brittle than the adult bone, so that unique fracture patterns different than that seen in adults, occur:

1. Plastic deformation - a bend in the bone without a fracture.
2. Green stick fracture - a fracture of one cortex under tension while the contralateral cortex remains intact.
3. Torus fracture - a fracture with buckling of one cortex in compression while the ocntralateral cortex is undamaged.

B. Bone Healing
Healing after a fracture in children is characterized by: rapidity, rare nonunion, and good remodeling potential. However, growth plate disturbances are possible which may cause late deformity.

C. Growth Plate
Ligaments are stronger than bone or growth plate in children. Thus, dislocations and sprains are relatively uncommon, while growth plate disruption and bone avulsion are more common in children. Growth plate injuries are described using the Salter-Harris classification. (see Musculoskeletal Disorders chapter)

II. EVALUATION OF MUSCULOSKELETAL SYSTEM

A. History
If the victim is conscious, a history is obtained to localize sites of pain.

B. Neurologic Examination
1. Nerve injury classification
    a) Neuropraxia - a physiologic but not anatomic disruption.
    b) Axonotmesis - axonal disruption, but not complete transection.
    c) Neurotmesis - complete nerve transection.

2. Common sites of nerve injury
    a) Posterior hip dislocation
    b) Distal humerus fracture
    c) Severe shoulder injuries usually correlate with amount of bone displacement

3. Rapid neurologic exam method
    A rapid neurologic examination is focused on motor strength including active flexion and extension of each major joint. Sensation should at least be tested on the dorsal and volar surfaces of each limb segment.

C. Skeletal Examination
The cervical spine must remain immobilized until fracture is ruled out. The spine is palpated for tenderness and deformity. Pelvic stability is assessed by lateral compression. The extremities are examined for tenderness, swelling and ecchymoses as signs of possible fractures or dislocations. In the absence of obvious fractures, passive flexion and extension can be performed on all extremities, and the long bones felt for creptius.

D. Vascular Examination
Vascular integrity must be ensured in every patient with musculoskeletal trauma. Fractures and dislocations around the elbow and knee are especially susceptible to vascular injury because arteries are tethered to bones at these sites. Poor peripheral pulses and slow capillary refill suggest vascular injury. Pain on passive stretch and tense swelling in a fascial compartment in addition to signs of vascular insufficiency suggest acute compartment syndrome.

E. X-rays
Areas indicated by abnormal physical findings (swelling, displacement, etc.) should be x-rayed. Specialized studies (computerized tomography, magnetic resonance imaging, or angiography) are obtained after consultation with an orthopedic surgeon. Orthopaedic surgery should be called early to help coordinate proper imaging and management. Patients sent to x-ray should have the extremety protected by splints until a fracture is ruled out.

III. COMPARTMENT SYNDROME (CS)

A. Mechanism of Injury: This syndrome develops because of increased compartment contents in a limiting fascial envelope. Increased contents can be from hemorrhage and cellular swelling from ischemia or blunt trauma. When compartment pressure is greater than capillary perfusion pressure, ischemia further complicates/aggravates compartment swelling. Obvious sequalae included distal vascular and neuro problems.

B. Evaluation
Clinical signs of CS described as the "5 P's":
1. Pain is out of proportion to that expected. The most sensitive finding in the physical exam is exquisite pain with passive stretch of the involved muscles.
2. Parethesia arises from sensory nerves contained in the compartment.
3. Pallor occurs in the distal part of the extremity due to poor capillary refill (> 3 seconds).
4. Pulselessness in the distal extremity is a very late sign.
5. Paralysis is also a late sign; early weakness should be sought instead.

CS is suspected even if only one of the above findings is present. Assessment relies on the accurate measurement of compartment pressure.

TREATMENT: Fasciotomy

IV.   **OPEN FRACTURES**

     A.   Cultures should be obtained from the would as soon as possible on presentation in the emergency room.

     B.   Antibiotic therapy: Include antistaphycoccal coverage (eg: a cephalosporin).

     C.   For severely contaminated, massive crush - or farm injuries: Add gentamicin and penicillin for Gram negative rod and streptococcal coverage.

     D.   Early operative debridement and irrigation is indicated in most cases, within 6 hours of injury.

     E.   Tetanus prophylaxis

V.   **REIMPLANTATION OF AMPUTATED EXTREMITY**

     A.   Rarely attempted for leg amputation, unless very "clean."

     B.   May be attempted in clean hand/arm cases.

     C.   Do not pack the amputated extremity directly on ice, rather it should be protected in a plastic bag, then cooled.

CHILDHOOD POISONINGS AND INGESTIONS

Jefry L. Biehler

Developmental Considerations

Poisonings and drug overdoses are common problems encountered by physicians caring for children. It is estimated that approximately 1.5 to 3 million poisonings occur in the United States each year. Sixty percent of these poisonings occur in children under the age of 5.

The optimum management of the poisoned or overdosed patient requires an organized approach of evaluation and treatment. This management should always focus on the patient first and the poison second. The stabilization of vital signs, including the establishment and maintenance of the ABC's (airway, breathing, circulation) is the first priority in all poisoned patients. This should be followed by an attempt to identify the responsible toxin, specific therapy if warranted, decontamination if indicated, and appropriate ongoing treatment or observation.

Diagnostic Modalities

Patient History and Physical Examination

A majority of patients (including pediatric patients) will present for evaluation or treatment with the ingestion of a known toxic substance. For these patients the identification of the toxin and suggested management strategies may be found in numerous texts and widely available computer based systems. For those patients presenting with an unknown ingestion or toxic exposure the history, physical examination, and proper laboratory tests frequently enables the physician to correctly identify the substance and provide necessary medical treatment.

If the patient is able to answer questions the physician should direct the history toward the identification of the ingested substance. An attempt to quantify the amount of toxic exposure, the elapsed time since exposure, and the development of symptoms since exposure should be elicited. For pediatric patients, available caretakers should be questioned. Questions should address the presence of household medications (prescription, over-the-counter and elicit drugs), other potential household toxins (cleaning compounds, plants, etc.), and possible environmental exposures (insecticides, herbicides, fertilizers).

Toxidromes

A combination of findings from a careful history and physical examination may allow physicians to clinically classify toxic ingestions into one of the common autonomic syndromes. These autonomic syndromes are often referred to as "Toxidromes" may be used as a basis for empiric treatment of ingestions prior to laboratory identification of specific toxins.

The four most commonly recognized Toxidromes are listed below:

Sympathomimetic Syndrome

Physical examination findings and symptoms

> Blood pressure elevated
> Heart rate elevated (except with severe hypertension)
> Pupils dilated
> Sweating
> Mental status changes (confused, anxious)
> Agitated
> Elevated temperature

Common substance ingestions associated with the sympathomimetic syndrome

> Cocaine
> Amphetamines
> PCP
> Phenylpropanolamine

Sympatholytic Syndrome

Physical examination findings and symptoms
        Blood pressure elevation
        Bradycardia
        Small pupils
        Mental status changes (obtunded, comatose)
        Decreased body temperature
        Decreased intestinal peristlsis

Common substance ingestions associated with the sympatholytic syndrome
        Ethanol
        Barbiturated
        Sedative-hypnotics
        Clonidine
        Opioids

Cholinergic Syndrome

Physical examination findings and symptoms associated
with the stimulation of Muscarinic receptors

S	Salivation (and Bronchorrhea)
L	Lacrimation
U	Urination
D	Diaphoresis
G	Gastrointestinal hyperperistalsis
E	Excitement (CNS) [from seizures to coma]
D	Decreased pupils, heart rate

Physical examination findings and symptoms associated
with the stimulation of Nicotinic receptors
        Initial hypertension and tachycardia
        Fasciculations and muscle weakness

Common substance ingestions associated with the cholinergic syndrome
        Organophosphates
        Carbamates
        Physostigmine
        Nicotine

Anticholinergic Syndrome

Physical examination findings and symptoms

Tachycardia
Hypertension
Elevated temperature
Dilated Pupils
Flushed, hot, dry skin
Decreased intestinal peristalsis
Urinary retention
Myoclonic jerking
Choreoathetoid movements
Mental status changes (agitated delirium)

Common substance ingestions associated with the anticohoinergic syndrome

Antihistamines
Cyclic antidepressants
Atropine
Scopolamine
Phenothiazines

Odor identification

Occasionally the identification of an ingested toxic substance is facilitated by the characteristic odor associated with the substance. The sensitivity of this method of toxin identification is very dependent on the observer. The following are some odors caused by toxins and drugs.

1. Acetone   Cholroform, Diabetic Ketoacidosis
2. Bitter almonds   Cyanide
3. Garlic   Arsenic, organophosphates
4. Mothballs   Naphthalene
5. Wintergreen   Methyl salicylate

Laboratory

Urine drug screening is often a useful tool in determining the presence of a specific ingested substance. However many authorities argue that the routine use of these screens without regard to available clinical and historical patient information is inefficient method of patient management. Toxidrome-oriented drug screening is a more cost and time efficient utilization of toxicologic testing.

The **Anion Gap** is another laboratory measurement utilized in the evaluation of poisoned patients. The Anion gap is calculated as follows:

$$Anion\ Gap = [Na] - ([HCO3] + [Cl])$$

$$Normal\ Anion\ Gap = 8 - 12$$

The anion gap is a method of quantifing the presence of anions not measure by routine laboratory tests. A patient with metabolic acidosis may therefore be further described as having an elevated, normal, or reduced anion gap.

A simple way of remembering the common drugs or poisons causing an elevated anion gap is using the phrase AT MUD PILES.

A	Alcohols
T	Toluene
M	Methanol
U	Uremia
D	DKA (Ketoacidosis)
P	Paraldehyde
I	Isoniazid, Iron, Ibuprofen
L	Lactic acid
E	Ethylene glycol
S	Salicylates

Another commonly measured "gap" in the evaluation of poisoned or overdosed patients is the osmolar gap. Serum osmolality may be measured in the laboratory by one of two methods. The first method utilizes the freezing point depression osmometer to determine osmolality. The second method uses a heat of vaporization method to determine osmolality. When measuring serum osmolality in the poisoned patient it is advisable to utilize the freezing point method. Alcohols may "boil off" before the serum osmolality is determined if the heat of vaporization method is used, thus giving a falsely normal osmolar gap.

Calc. Osmolality = 2[Na] + [glucose]/2 + [BUN]/2.8 = 285-295 mosm/L

Osmolar gap = measured - calculated osmolality

A simple way of remembering the common drugs or poisons causing an elevated osmolar gap is using the phrase MEAN PIE.

M	Mannitol, Mehtanol
E	Ethanol, Ethyl ether
A	Acetone
N	"No Kidneys" (Renal failure without dialysis
P	Propylene glycol
I	Isopropyl alcohol
E	Ethylene glycol

X-ray identification

Abdominal x-rays may reveal radiopaque ingested substances. Recently ingested iron containing tablets may be seen on plain x- rays. The sensitivity of this method for determining the presence of ingested materials is to low to make this a routine part of the evaluation of poisoned patients.

Theraputic Considerations

DECONTAMINATION

The process of decontamination is usually divided into three areas 1) decontamination of the eyes, 2) decontamination of the skin, 3) gastrointestinal decontamination.

Skin decontamination:

Because many toxins are rapidly absorbed through the skin (ie organophosphates) the removal of these substances from the skin surface should be undertake expeditiouly. Contaminated clothing should be removed and the contaminated skin flushed with large amounts of water or saline. Care must be taken to avoid exposure to health care personel during the decontamination process.

Eye decontamination:

Large volumes of warm water or saline should be used to flush the eyes of persons with toxic exposure of the eyes.

Gastrointestinal decontamination:

There is an ongoing controversy regarding the use of gastric decontamination in the poisoned patient. Many authors feel that the use of induced emesis or gastric lavage is only minimally effective in reducing the dosage of ingested substances. Many authors feel that the use of activated charcoal without prior gastric emptying is a more effective method of gastrointestinal decontamination. However the routine use of induced emesis and gastric lavage is still a common practice among physicians caring for overdosed patients.

Induced Emesis

The most common method of inducing emesis in the overdosed/poisoned patient is the adminstration of syrup of ipecac. This medication acts by both direct gastric mucosal irritation and by effects on the central nervous system. Although not recommended by most authors, apomorphine, an opiate derivative, is also effective in inducing emesis.

Contraindications for inducing emesis in poisoned patients are as follows:

1. Patients in a coma or depressed neurologic condition
2. Patients who have ingested substances which may result in sudden deterioration of mental status
3. Patients with a depressed or absent gag reflex
4. Patients who are have seizures
5. Patients who have ingested caustics
6. Patients who have ingested hydrocarbons

Gastric Lavage

Gastric lavage with a large-bore nasogastric or orogastric tube is probalby slightly more effective at removing ingested substances than induced emesis. The complications associated with this method of decontamination are listed below:

1. Perforation of the esophagus or stomach
2. Aspiration of stomach contents during placement
3. Inadvertent tracheal intubation with the gastric tube
4. Trauma to the nares or oral mucosa during placement
5. Patient discomfort during tube placement

Activated charcoal

The administration of activated charcoal as a liquid slurry is an effective method of intestinal decontamination. Activated charcoal is very adsorbent of most common poisons and drugs. The large surface area produced in the activation process allows the charcoal to absorb significant amounts of ingested substances. Charcoal is indicated in almost all ingestions. Although some substances are poorly adsorbed by activated charcoal (iron, lithium, cyanide, alcohols, acids and bases) the potential advantageous effects outweith potential risks. The contraindications for the adminstration of charcoal are listed below:

1. Patients who are to undergo endoscopy for manual removal of ingested substances.
2. Patients with ileus or intestinal obstruction

Cathartics

Cathartics are used to hasten the elimination of poisons or ingested substances from the gastrointestinal tract. Substances used to decrease gastrointestinal transit times include the following: 1) magnesium citrate, 2) sorbitol, and 3) polyethylene glycol solutions. The contraindications for cathartic administration are listed below:

1. Patients with ileus or intestinal obstruction
2. Comatose, convulsing or obtunded patients

Specific Indications for hemodialysis

Lithium	> 4.0 mEq/L
Salicylates	> 100 mg/dl
Methanol	> 50 mg/dl
Ethylene glycol	> 50 mg/dl

A number of specific antidotes are available for the treatment of selected toxins.

Toxin	Antidote
Acetaminophen	N-acetylcysteine
Atropine	Physostigmine
Arsenic	Dimercaprol
Benzodiazipines	Flumazonil
Carbon monoxide	Oxygen
Digoxin	Digitalis antibodies
Ethylene glycol	Ethanol
Heparin	Protamine
Iron	Deferoxamine mesylate
Lead	EDTA
Mercury	Dimercaprol
Methanol	Ethanol
Nitrates	Methylene Blue
Opiates	Naloxone
Organophosphates	Pralidoxime
Zinc	EDTA

Potentially toxic acute doses of selected poisons

Toxin	Potentially toxic ingestion	Lethal ingestion
Acetominophen	150 mg/kg	
Iron	> 60 mg/kg	
Salicylates	100 mg/kg	
Ethylene Glycol		1-1.5 ml/kg
Methanol		0.5 ml/kg

Nancy R. Inhofe

Sexual Abuse of Children

I. GENERAL CONSIDERATIONS
    A. Definition of Sexual Abuse
        1. The involvement of a child in sexual activities that the child cannot comprehend, for which the child is developmentally unprepared and cannot give informed consent, and/or that violate the social and legal taboos of society.
        2. Acts range from indecent exposure and pornography to physical contact. Contact exposure may include touching, or fondling through clothes, direct touching or fondling of the genitals, simulated intercourse or vulva-coitus, coitus, sodomy, oral sex, instrumentation.
        3. Activities occur between 2 or more people of discrepant ages (4-5 years) for the sexual gratification of the older person.

II. ETIOLOGY
    A. Several theories exist to provide a model for understanding how sexual abuse of children occurs. Finklehor describes "four preconditions of sexual abuse".
        1. Motivation to sexual abuse
            a. Emotional congruence
            b. Sexual arousal
            c. Individual's inability to have normal sexual relationships
            d. Experience as a sexually abused child
        2. Internal inhibitors
            a. Alcohol and drugs are the two most common destroyers of normal inhibitors
        3. Overcoming external inhibitors
            a. Presence of a protective parent
        4. Breakdown of the child's resistance
            a. Factors that decrease resistance include: cohersion, fear, developmental immaturity, retardation

III. DEVELOPMENTAL CONSIDERATIONS
    A. Most newborn female infants have some white vaginal discharge: 10-15% will have vaginal bleeding due to estrogen withdrawal. These vaginal secretions usually disappear within 2-3 weeks. Persistence of vaginal bleeding beyond 4-6 weeks is unusual and deserves evaluation.
        1. In prepubertal girls, the pH of the vagina is alkaline rather than acid.
        2. Prepubertal female children are generally examined externally for signs of sexual abuse. A speculum exam is not recommended. In cases of vaginal bleeding from an unknown site or foreign body, an exam should be done under anesthesia.

3. The uterus and adnexal areas may be palpated more readily with a rectal exam than vaginal exam due to the short posterior fornix.

4. If the clinical signs of puberty develop prior to age 8 in the female or prior to age 9 in the male, is termed precocious.

5. Following maternal estrogen withdrawal, the labia minora becomes lined with non-stratified squamous epithelium. In response to trauma or inflammation, the adjacent surfaces of the labia minora may agglutinate and become adherent. This is known as labial adhesions. These are common and produce few symptoms. They are not thought to be indicative of sexual abuse.

B. Development of sexuality in preschool children
1. These children commonly wonder where babies come from.
2. Some are interested in physical differences between boys and girls. By the end of the preschool years, most children are aware of the sex-role differences.
3. Occasional masturbation is quite frequent.
4. Concern about sexual intercourse or other forms of adult sexual behavior is rare in children who have not been involved in or exposed to such behaviors.
5. Masturbation and playing doctor or other exploratory games with friends and siblings is seen between the ages of 4 and 6.
6. Some flirtatious behavior may be normal, though it is generally reserved for the familiar opposite sex parent. If the behavior is indiscriminate, the possibility of sexual abuse must be considered.
7. Between the ages of 6 and 12, there is a decrease in sex play.

IV. INDICATORS OF SEXUAL ABUSE
A. Allegations disclosed by the child
1. Only about 20% of children eventually diagnosed as being abused.
2. Sexually abused present with the chief complaint of abuse.
3. Sexual abuse to a physician.
B. Non-specific genito-urinary and anal complaints
1. Irritation or pain
2. Discharge
3. Bleeding
4. Frequent urinary tract infections
C. Pregnancy
D. Sexually transmitted diseases
1. Niceria gonorrhea (Ng)
   a. Organism
      1. Aerobic gram negative diplococci
      2. In vitro requires free iron, CO_2
      3. Ng morphologically similar to other species of the Neisseria genus

          4.   Incubation period 2 - 7 days

   b.   Clinical features of infection

        1.   Vaginal

            i.   Up to 44% asymptomatic for up to 6 months

            ii.   Vulvovaginitis: profuse green discharge, erythema, edema, pruritus, pyuria and dysuria

        2.   Urethral

            i.   Urethral erythema, discharge, pruritus, testicular swelling, balanitis, inguinal adenopathy

        3.   Rectal

            i.   Most asymptomatic

        4.   Pharyngeal

            i.   Only 25% symptomatic

        5.   Systemic and ascending manifestations

            i.   Rare prior to puberty

            ii.   Peritonitis, PID, arthritis, sepsis

   c.   Diagnosis

        1.   Gram stain: gram negative intracellular diplococci

            i.   Sensitivity: -50%

            ii.   Highly specific in prepubertal children

        2.   Culture from all 3 sites (vaginal, not cervical)

            i.   Inoculate appropriate culture media at room temperature

            ii.   Confirmatory testing by 2 independent methods to rule out false positive result

        3.   Store isolates at -70^0C

            i.   May compare patient's isolate with suspect's isolate (auxotype and serovar)

   d.   Transmission

        1.   Sexual contact

            i.   Confirmed culture from any site represents sexual transmission

        2.   Vertical transmission from infected mother

            i.   Ophthalmia neonatorum, rectal and nasopharyngeal infection; disseminated disease

        3.   Fomites: No evidence

   e.   Implication

        1.   Sexual abuse is medical certainty even without a history or other physical indicators

2.   Chlamydia Trachomatis (Ct)

   a.   Organism

        1.   Obligate intracellular bacterial parasite

        2.   Most prevalent STD in adults and children

  b.   Clinical features of infection

        1.   Vaginal infection

              i.   75% asymptomatic

              ii.   Mild vulvovaginitis possibly due to another pathogen

        2.   Urethritis

        3.   Rectal: usually asymptomatic

        4.   Pharyngeal infection rare

  c.   Diagnosis

        1.   Culture of vagina, urethra, rectum is GOLD STANDARD

              i.   Best swab type: Dacron on aluminum

              ii.   Good recovery of isolates if 4^0C for 24 hours or freeze at -70^0C.

        2.   Non-culture methods not approved

              i.   Low prevalence group

              ii.   Cross reactivity with other flora

              iii.   Cannot store isolates

  d.   Transmission

        1.   Sexual contact

               i.   Mucosal contact or genital secretions on hands

              ii.   Reported rates in abused children 4-17% for vaginal and rectal infection

              iii.   Few valid control groups comparing rates of Ct infection in children (abused vs. nonabused)

        2.   Vertical transmission

               i.   Delivery through infected cervix or prolonged rupture of membranes

              ii.   15% born to culture positive women acquire rectal or vaginal infection

              iii.   Infection may be asymptomatic and persistent up to 3 years after birth. Duration is uncertain

        3.   Fomites

               i.   No evidence for genital strains

  e.   Implication

        1.   Probable indicator of sexual abuse (AAP)

        2.   ? Ct in genital tract at any age warrants investigation

3.   Condyloma Acuminata

  a.   Organism

        1.   Human papilloma virus (HPV)

               i.   DNA virus, group A papovavirus

              ii.   >50 known types

        2.   Types associated with anatomic location

               i.   Genital types: 6, 11, 16, 18, 31, 35

           ii.   Laryngeal types: 6, 11

           iii.   Skin types: 1-4

    3.   Oncogenic types: 16, 18, 31

    4.   Prolonged incubation or latency period (1-20 months) makes source difficult to identify

b.   Clinical features of infection

    1.   Variable appearance: Soft papillary or verrucous growths on skin or mucous membranes

    2.   Subclinical: visible with 3-5% acetic acid and magnification

    3.   Associated with bleeding, pain, difficult defecation, other STDs

c.   Diagnosis

    1.   Clinical appearance

    2.   Biopsy and histopathology

    3.   Southern blot for type

           i.   May exclude an alleged perpetrator

           ii.   Identify those at risk for later malignancy

d.   Transmission

    1.   Sexual contact

           i.   Lesions develop in 60% of sexual partners

    2.   Vertical transmission

           i.   Infants acquire laryngeal, anal, genital warts

           ii.   Transplacental vs. birth canal

e.   Close contact and autoinoculation

    1.   Not known whether genital types transmitted by non-veneral means

f.   Implication

    1.   Probable indicator of sexual abuse

           i.   25-80% reported cases confirmed due to sexual abuse

           ii.   Known case reports of sexual abuse in children with genital HPV whose mother had similar lesions and no other apparent risks, and in children with skin warts

4.   Trichomonas Vaginalis

a.   Organism

    1.   Flagellate protozoan

    2.   Acid pH, moist conditions

    3.   Prevalence: 20-30% adult females, unknown in children

b.   Clinical features of infection

    1.   Vaginal

           i.   Vaginitis: odorous, green discharge, vaginal erythema

           ii.   Present in 3-5% asymptomatic women

    2.   Urethral: all men asymptomatic

        c.   Diagnosis

             1.   Wet prep

                  i.   Motile flagellated organism slightly larger than a WBC

                  ii.   Sensitivity only 50%

             2.   Culture

                  i.   Expensive

                  ii.   Not readily available

        d.   Transmission

             1.   Sexual contact

             2.   Vertical transmission

                  i.   Persists in vagina up to one year

    5.   Other STDs

        a.   Syphilis (Treponema pallidum)

             1.   Diagnosis by serology

             2.   Need follow-up in 6-12 weeks

             3.   In 1990, consensus for routine testing

             4.   Definite indicator of sexual abuse if not acquired perinatally

        b.   Herpes Simplex Virus I and II

             1.   Diagnose by culture

             2.   Transmission

                  i.   Sexual contact

                  ii.   Perinatal-up to 30 days after birth

                  iii.   Autoinoculation documented for both types

                  iv.   Fomites: not documented

             3.   Implication of genital lesions

                  i.   Type II probable indicator

                  ii.   Type I possible indicator

        c.   HIV

             1.   HIV transmission through sexual abuse in 4 of 96 children (Duke University, <u>AJDC</u>, Feb. 1991)

             2.   Consensus of 63 experts for screening

                  i.   Consensus:

<u>Victim</u>	<u>Assailant</u>
1. Clinical profile AIDS/ARC	1. HIV seropositive
2. Behavioral high risk (prostitute, homosexual, drugs)	2. Clinical profile AIDS/ARC
3. Parent/adolescent insistence	3. Behavioral high risk
	4. Multiple assailants

        d.   Bacterial Vaginosis

             1.   Not a marker for sexual activity

             2.   Major mode of acquisition probably not sexual

E.   Atypical, recurrent physical complaints
1.   Neurologic (Dizziness, weakness, headaches)
2.   Abdominal pain
3.   Chest pain
F.   Behavioral Signs
1.   Sleeping disturbances
2.   Change in appetite
3.   School problems
4.   Regressive behaviors
5.   Running away from home
6.   Alcohol/drug abuse
7.   Sexual acting out and excessive sexual knowledge
8.   Change in affect including fear, anger, depression
G.   Physical Signs
1.   Bruises, scratches, bites
2.   Blood stains on underwear
3.   Bruising, swelling of genital area, not consistent with history
4.   Injury to lips
5.   Grasp marks

V.   DIAGNOSTIC PLAN
A.   The interview
1.   The interview remains the most critical factor in establishing whether or not sexual abuse has occurred.
2.   Interviewer should be skilled at taking a history in a non-leading fashion, with the ability to show no embarrassment to the child, and with a sensitive, non-aggressive approach.
3.   Documentation of the interview using first person in quotations is preferable.
B.   Behavioral Assessment
C.   Medical Exam
1.   Purpose
    a.   Reassure the child and family
    b.   Treat medical conditions
    c.   Legal interaction
2.   Technique
    a.   a general examination is done to note the child's Tanner Stage of development, the child's affect and any evidence of extra-genital trauma or dermatitis.
    b.   Genital and anal examination is done in frog-leg, prone knee/chest, or lithotomy (stirrup) positions and labial separation or traction is done to separate the labia majora in order to have a good field of vision.
    c.   A good light source and magnification can be obtained through colposcopy.
    d.   All perineal structures should be described using the face of a clock

for positions. Careful attention to the clitoris and prepuce, urethra, apari-urethral areas, peri-hymenal tissue, hymen, vestibule (fossa navicularis), posterior fourchette, median raphe, anus with rugal folds, tone and wink noted.

    e.   Hymen should be described as redundant or fimbriated, annular, crescentic.

    f.   Hymenal tissue should be evaluated, the size of the hymenal opening is difficult to obtain and varies with the child's age, relaxation, and labial separation techniques.

    g.   Abnormal hymenal os dimensions should not be used alone as physical evidence of abuse.

    h.   Avoid using terms such as hymen intact, virginal, ruptured.

D.   Common Terminology used to describe abnormalities include:
    1.   Hyperemia or erythema, scarring, adhesions, transection, attenuation, key-hole deformity

E.   Cultures
    1.   Oral pharynx, vagina or urethra and rectum for gonorrhea
    2.   Cultures should be done from the rectum and vagina for chlamydia. (I will include a chart from the CDC's recommendations.)

F.   Documentation
    1.   Documentation of findings should be accurate. May use description in text form, trauma gram, photographs.

THE INTERVIEW REMAINS THE MOST CRITICAL FACTOR IN ESTABLISHING WHETHER OR NOT SEXUAL ABUSE HAS OCCURRED.

A.   General comments
    1.   Lack of embarrassment
    2.   Concept of touch
    3.   Do not solely use words "pain", "hurt"
    4.   Avoid leading questions
    5.   Children may feel anxious, fearful, guilty
    6.   Ask Who, Where, What questions
        a.   "Why" questions are difficult for children
    7.   Neutral setting
        a.   Talk to child separate from the caretaker
    8.   Avoid multiple interviewers
    9.   Child's age
        a.   Use child's terminology

b.   Use child's sense of time

   10. Determine continuum of perpetrator acts

B.   Documenting the interview

     1.   Identify accompanying adult, primary caretaker, and perpetrator by name in full, address, phone if possible

     2.   <u>Who</u> did <u>What</u>, <u>How Often</u>, <u>Where</u>, <u>When</u>

     3.   Record child's own words

          a.   Use first person in quotations

          b.   Statements may be admissable if in record

     4.   Time elapsed between suspected abuse and statement

     5.   Whether spontaneous or in response to a questions

     6.   Whether spontaneous or from reflective thought

     7.   If in response to leading or non-leading questions

     8.   Observe signs of excitement/distress (excited utterances)

     9.   Physical condition at time of statement

     10.   Who present when statement was made, where it was made, when, and to whom

C.   Past medical history

     1.   Genitourinary complaints

          a.   Recurrent UTIs

          b.   Vaginal bleeding, infection, discharge

          c.   Pregnancy

     2.   Age of menses, LMP, use of tampons

     3.   Stooling pattern

     4.   Birth control

     5.   Previous abuse

     6.   Skin disorders

     7.   Bleeding diathesis

     8.   Maternal STD and mode of delivery

     9.   Developmental history in younger children

          a.   Age of walking, toilet training

          b.   Regressive behavior (enuresis)

D.   Behavioral assessment

     1.   Victims often develop age and situation related behavior disturbances

          a.   School refusal

          b.   Sleep disturbances

          c.   Excessive masturbation

          d.   Sexually provocative behavior

          e.   Fear/anxiety

     2.   In older children

          a.   School failure

          b.   Promiscuity

          c.   Runaway

            d.   Drug/alcohol abuse
            e.   Suicide
            f.   Eating disorders
            g.   Depression
2.   The Medical examination
        A.   Purpose
                1.   Reassure the child and family
                2.   Treat medical conditions (STD)
                3.   Legal interaction
        B.   General comments
                1.   Avoid further trauma to the child
                        a.   Explain exam to the child
                        b.   May have supportive, familiar adult present
                        c.   Conduct as part of a general physical exam
                2.   Problems regarding the medical examination
                        a.   Lack of formal physician training
                        b.   Range of normal variants
                        c.   Most exams normal due to nature of abuse

        C.   Forensic examination
                1.   Perform exam immediately if abuse occurred within 72 hours
                        a.   Rape kit protocols for "chain of evidence"
                2.   Assault more than 72 hours prior to visit
                        a.   May schedule elective exam

        D.   Technique
                1.   General examination
                        a.   Note Tanner stage of development
                        b.   Note the child's affect
                        c.   Note evidence of extragenital trauma or dermatitis
                2.   Genital/anal examination
                        a.   Positioning (see Diagram 1)
                                1.   Frogleg, knee-chest, or lithotomy
                                2.   Labial separation and traction
                        b.   Normal anatomy
                                1.   Describe all structures (see Diagram 2)
                                        a.   Use "face of clock"
                                2.   Hymenal description (Pokorny)
                                        a.   Three categories (amount and distribution of tissue)
                                                1.   Fimbriated
                                                2.   Annular
                                                3.   Crescentic
                                        b.   Note size of hymenal opening
                                        c.   Evaluate tissue

        c.   Terminology
- 1. Hyperemia
- 2. Scar
- 3. Synechiae
- 4. Transection
- 5. Attenuation
- 6. Key-hole deformity
- 7. Notches and bumps

        d.   Colposcopy: used externally for magnification (5-30x) and light source

        e.   Culture techniques (see STD)

        f.   Accurate documentation
- 1. Use traumagram
- 2. Describe in text
- 3. Photographs

E. Medical findings and interpretation
- 1. Acute and chronic findings
  - a. Acute
    - 1. Usually no findings
    - 2. Erythema
    - 3. Contusions
    - 4. Abrasions
    - 5. Edema
    - 6. Lacerations
  - b. Chronic
    - 1. Usually no findings
    - 2. Rarely-healed transections
  - c. Findings more often in the anterior 180 degrees of hymen
- 2. Digital penetration
  - a. Acute
    - 1. Abrasions
    - 2. Lacerations of lateral and ventral hymen
  - b. Chronic
    - 1. Healed transections
  - c. Findings more often in the anterior 180 degrees of hymen, clitoris
- 3. Vulvar intercourse
  - a. Acute
    - 1. Abrasions
    - 2. Lacerations
    - 3. Bruising
  - b. Chronic
    - 1. Scarring of introitus or vestibular mucosa
- 4. Vaginal penetration

a. Acute
1. Abrasions, lacerations, bruising
2. Muscle spasm
3. Semen
b. Chronic
1. Distorted, asymmetric, thickened, rounded or scalloped hymenal tissue
2. Rounded hymenal remnants
3. Scars more often in posterior 180 degrees of hymen, fossa navicularis and posterior fourchette
4. May be no findings (David Muram)
5. Anal penetration
a. Acute
1. Sphincter initially relaxed, then in spasm
2. Edema of anal verge
3. Erythema
4. Abrasions, bruised, tears
5. Semen
b. Chronic
1. Relaxed tone or inhibited wink
2. Thickened rugal folds
3. Coving
4. Scars-fanshaped or linear
5. Skin tags
c. May be no findings
1. Extent of findings depend on
a. Size/shape of object
b. Age/size of child
c. Use of lubrication
d. Force of entry
6. Penile trauma
a. Acute
1. None
2. Lacerations, bruises, bite marks
3. Urethral damage, discharge
b. Chronic
1. Telangiectasia

F. Interpretation
1. A normal examination should not be used to rule out sexual abuse
2. Measuring hymenal dimensions
a. Difficult to obtain
b. Varies with child's age, relaxation, labial separation techniques
c. Should not be used alone as physical evidence of abuse

3. THE HISTORY SHOULD BE CONSISTENT WITH THE NATURE AND DEGREE OF THE INJURIES

4. Rules of thumb

    a. Subtle findings are suggestive but not diagnostic of sexual abuse

    b. Dating of injuries more than 1-2 weeks old is <u>not</u> possible

    c. Acute injuries heal rapidly and most do not leave persistent signs of trauma

    d. Most sexual abuse victims have normal exams

3. Laboratory examination

    A. STD (see STD outline III.)

    B. Non-venereal causes of Vulvovaginitis and Proctitis

        1. Foreign body

        2. Chemical irritation

        3. Infections

            a. Candida

            b. Beta hemolytic streptococci

            c. Shigella

            d. Yersinia

        4. Bleeding diathesis

        5. Pregnancy

VI. Differential diagnosis of possible sexual abuse

1. Vulvovaginitis

2. Foreign body

3. Dermatitis (seborrhea, lichen sclerosis)

4. Behcet's

5. Labial adhesions (agglutination)

6. Accidental trauma/straddle injuries or previous surgical or invasive medical procedures

7. Failure of midline fusion

8. Prominent median raphe

9. Infection (non-STD): Group A Strep Shigella

10. Septate hymen

11. Urethral prolapse

VII. Treatment and follow-up

    A. Treat and test for cure of STD

        1. Prophylaxis after initial exam

            a. Assailant known to be infected

            b. Follow-up of victim unlikely

            c. Ceftriaxone IM and Doxycycline or EES po

        2. Specific regimens: See CDC recommendations

    B. Pregnancy test 2 weeks post assault

        1. Pregnancy prophylaxis if within 48 hours of assault

C.   Syphilis serology 6 weeks post assault
D.   HIV 3 and 6 months post assault
E.   Referrals to Social Services, Child Protective Services (CPS), psychological evaluation and counseling
F.   **REASSURE THE CHILD**
G.   **PREVENTIVE COUNSELING**

VIII.   Prognosis
A.   Prognosis is highly variable and is largely dependent on early psychotherapy for both the child and the non-offending caretakers.
B.   Prevention is better than treatment.
C.   Poor self-esteem, depression, guilt, suicidal gestures, acting sexually inappropriate or excessive preoccupation with masturbation, delinquency, running away, substance abuse, prostitution, nd psychosomatic gynecological and gastrointestinal complaints.

IX.   Legal issues
A.   Mandatory reporting of "suspected" abuse by any physician. Abuse does not have to be proven in order to make a report to Child Protective Services (CPS).
1.   Required in all states
2.   Penalties for failure to report
3.   Medical liability risks
a.   Not recognizing sexual abuse in a timely manner
b.   Unsubstantiated reports
1.   Statutes give immunity if reporting done in good faith
B.   Adjudication in juvenile court
1.   Deprived status
2.   "Preponderance of evidence"
3.   Best interest of child and family
C.   Adjudication in criminal court
1.   "Beyond a reasonable doubt"
2.   Focus on substantiation of criminal act by accused perpetrator
D.   Divorce/custody proceedings
1.   Increasing numbers
2.   Do not dismiss because of custody dispute

X.   Conclusions
A.   State final impression in terms of clinical findings
1.   History
2.   Physical examination
3.   Behavioral indicators
B.   Examples of medical record assessment entry
1.   <u>Summary:</u>   Five-year-old female reports that her uncle touched her "bottom" with his fingers. The physical examination is normal and consistent with the history as given by the child.

Behavioral indicator of new onset enuresis could be indicative of environmental stress."

Conclusion: "Possible sexual abuse based on the history, a consistent physical examination and behavioral changes."

2. Summary: "Twelve-year-old female consistently reports painful penile-vaginal penetration over several years by her stepfather. Physical examination is consistent with blunt-force penetrating trauma of the vagina. Behavior changes are unknown at present."

Conclusion: "Sexual abuse based on history and physical examination."

XI. Importance of documentation
    A. Likelihood of CPS/legal involvement is high
        1. Keep detailed records, drawings, photographs
        2. Submit written reports to agencies
    B. The ability to protect a child may often depend on the quality of the physician's records

CHILD ABUSE

I. Physical Abuse
    A. General Considerations
        1. Definition
            a. Physical abuse is any non-accidental injury to a child under the age of 18 by a parent or caretaker. An injury is defined as any type of tissue injury including bruises, burns, fractures and internal injuries.
            b. Physical abuse is typically a pattern of behavior that is repeated over time but may also be a single physical attack.
        2. Incidence/Prevalence
            a. 675,000 confirmed cases per year in the U.S.
            b. Minimum of 3 children die per day as a result of physical abuse and neglect.
            c. 95% of child fatalities in <3 year olds. These figures likely underrepresent the actual incidence of abuse.
        3. Etiology
            a. The cause of physical abuse is complex and variable. It is most useful to understand child abuse as a symptom of a dysfunctional family. Both families and children are known to have characteristics of which place them at greater risk of child abuse.
                1. Vulnerable families

a. Socially isolated, domestic violence among the adults in the family, parents who were maltreated as children, substance abuse, mental illness.

2. Vulnerable children

a. Prematurity, birth to a young parent, genital abnormalities, or any condition that interferes with parent/child bonding.

3. Crisis situation

B. Developmental Considerations

1. Younger children more likely to be abused.

2. Developmental skills important to assessment.

a. Example includes: a month old who alledgely rolls off of dressing table and sustains serious head trauma; Note: a one month old does not roll front to back or back to front at this age.

b. Children who do not ambulate are unlikely to have burns on the soles of their feet.

C. Indicators

D. Diagnostic Approach

1. The medical history: Because there are few syndromes of inflicted injury, the medical history is of great importance in determining accidental versus inflicted injury.

a. An approach

1. Separate interviews from child and caretaker.

2. Tell the child and caretaker the reason for the interview.

3. Be supportive of both the child and parent.

4. Explain that physicians are mandated reporters of suspected child abuse.

b. Clues to possible abuse

1. Injury not consistent with the age or developmental ability of the child.

2. Triggering behavior of the child, for example: colic or toilet training failures.

3. Descrepant history (changing, vague, severity or pattern not consistent with the history of the injury)

4. Delay in seeking medical care.

5. Multiple hospitals or clinics used for medical care.

6. Crisis for abuser.

7. Social isolation.

8. No witness.

9. Withdrawn, submissive child and no appropriate parental affect.

10. History of abuse in the parent.

2. The medical examination-Physical injuries/Modes of presentation

a. Bruises

1. Shape or pattern: A bruise may resemble the shape of the object used to inflict the injury, eg., hand or finger-shaped bruises, belt buckles, electrical cords.

2. Location: Unintentional bruises most commonly involve the forehead, chin, cheekbone, shins, and forearms. Abdominal bruises are unusual. Genital bruises and peri-anal bruising is rarely unintentional.

3. Color/age: Multiple injuries of different ages is a hallmark of child abuse. Bruises resolve in a predictable pattern. (Will add a chart)

4. Child's age: Any injury of an infant (non-ambulatory) should be suspect for being an abusive injury.

5. Pathological condition: It is generally thought best to rule-out a coagulopathy when diffuse bruising is seen.

b. Burns

1. Agent

a. Hot liquids cause 75% of all burns. These burns are generally immersion in type.

b. Other common agents include hot objects (steam irons or curling irons), electrical, chemical, fire/flash burns.

2. Pattern

a. Immersion: Generally in a glove or pantyhose-like configuration with sparing of areas including the flection creases and fuse flashmarks from a child being forced and held in hot water.

b. Hot objects: Multiple, characteristically-shaped iron burns are rarely unintentional. Cigarette burns are usually confused with impetigo.

3. Severity

a. Depends on exposure, time, temperature, type of agent, thickness of skin. (Will need chart) NOTE: Most hot water heaters are set at 140^0F. At this water temperature, it takes 3 seconds for a first or second-degree burn and 15 seconds for a third-degree burn.

3. Fractures

a. Types

1. Specific for abuse, spiral fracture of the long bone in non-ambulating infants, metaphacial "corner" fractures (due to violent traction or rotation) and "bucket handle" fractures and rib fractures in less than 2 year olds (90% of rib fractures in children less than two are abuse-related. The rib cage is compliant and cannot be fractured in accidental falls

or CPR in children. Rib fractures are caused by a violent antero-posterior compression of the chest. 80% of rib fractures in children are clinically unsuspected).

2. Virtually diagnostic occult fractures inconsistent with a history and three or more fractures in various stages of healing and associated extra-skeletal injury.

3. Suspicious pariostial new-bone formation (bone bruise due to a traumatic separation by traction or tortion). Not specific to traumatic injury as maybe due to infection or metabolic disorders.

4. Exceptions: nursemaid's elbow, linear parietal skull fracture from a fall of three to four feet to a hard surface, toddler's fracture (spiral, non-displaced fracture of the tibia in ambulating toddlers require fixation of the extremity above and below the joint).

b. Age of child: Any fracture of a child less than two years of age is highly suspicious. 2/3 of these fractures are due to child abuse.

c. Pathological conditions

1. Osteogenesis imperfecta

2. Copper deficiency

3. Congenital syphilis, vitamin C and D deficiencies, Caffey's disease and paraplega or indifference to pain syndromes.

d. Healing pattern helps to date the time of injury

1. Pariostial new-bone 5-10 days

2. Soft callus 10-14 days

3. Hard callus 14-21 days

4. Head Trauma

a. Mechanism

1. Rotational: rapid acceleration and deceleration, shaking-type injury without impact.

2. Translational: impact may occur by hitting head-on inanimate object including walls or tables or by intentional closed fist.

3. Fall heights: it is unusual and has not been documented to have skull fracture falls less than 3-4 feet. An exception to this is the simple linear, non-thiostatic parietal skull fracture.

b. Patterns

1. Shaken Baby Sundrome

a. May be no external signs or skull fracture but intracranial hemorrhage and retinal hemorrhages are found. Occasionally, long bone fractures.

2. Skull Fracture Types found considerably more often in abused children include multiple or complex configuration; depressed, wide or growing fractures; involvement of more than one cranial bone; non-parietal fractures; and associated

intracranial injury; bilateral fractures; fractures crossing suture lines; diastatic fractures greater than or equal to 3 milimeters in width. NOTE: Suspicion is greatly enhanced when there is no history of trauma or when only a minor fall is reported.

       3.   Other markers

           1.   Extra-cranial injury including scalp, subgalial hemorrhages, hair-pulling injuries, retinal hemorrhaging.

           2.   Intracranial hemorrhage, contusion or edema.

           3.   Concurrent skeletal injuries (these are found in 70% of skull fractures from abuse)

           4.   Evidence of muscle injury from extracranial abuse include urine myoglobin and CPK.

    c.   Age of skull fractures in children less than 6 months of age are generally non-accidental. In addition, head trauma is the principle cause of morbidity and mortality in the child abuse syndrome.

    5.   Internal injuries

       a.   Visceral trauma

           1.   Generally occurs in children more than two years of age.

           2.   Blunt injury is more common than penetrating trauma.

           3.   Injuries generally occur to the abdominal structures that are fixed and may be crushed between the inflicting instrument and the rotibral bodies. These include the duodenum, musitary and pancreas.

           4.   Visceral trauma is usually occul, i.e., there is no external bruising.

       b.   Munchausen's by proxy

           1.   Definition

               a.   The intentional creation or description of an illness in a child by a parent who intends to involve the child in a continuing process of medical diagnosis and care.

           2.   Example: The parent who induces apnea by suffocation of the infant to the point of loss of consciousness or seizure.

           3.   The induced symptoms may lead to lethal outcome

       c.   Intentional intoxication includes the use of alcohol and sedative drugs in order to suppress undesirable childhood behaviors and to facilitate sexual abuse of the child.

II. DIAGNOSTIC MODALITIES

    A.   Radiologic imaging

       1.   Routine x-rays

           a.   Skeletal survey

               i.   Recommended in all children less than two years of age who have clinical evidence of physical abuse or neglect.

ii.　Includes frontal and lateral skull with lateral cervical spine, lateral thoracolumbar spine, frontal chest, frontal upper extremities and frontal lower extremities to include shoulder girdle, lower lumbar spine, pelvis, hands and feet.

2.　Cranial CT Scan

a.　Remains the primary cranio-cerebral imaging technique in investigation of inflicted intracranial trauma. Superior to MRI for subarachnoid hemorrhage, evaluation of calvarial injury and is more easily performed in the unstable patient.

3.　MRI

a.　Superior to CT in depicting deep cerebral injuries, determining the age of extracerebral fluid collections, including small subdural hematomas.

4.　Bone Scan

a.　Sensitive for acute non-displaced and subtle healing fractures.

b.　Insensitive for skull and vertebral body fractures.

B.　Retinal Exam

1.　Retinal hemorrhages are quite specific for the shaken infant syndrome.

2.　Retinal hemorrhages are also seen in approximately 15-20% of newborn infants but resolve within the first several weeks of life.

C.　CSF Exam

1.　Examthrochromic CSF outside of the immediate newborn indicates subarachnoid hemorrhage, generally due to trauma. This finding may be helpful in determining the cause of diminished level of consciousness in an infant presenting to the Emergency Department.

D.　Coagulation Studies

1.　PT, PTT, platelets, bleeding time, support the diagnosis of battered child syndrome as opposed to coagulopathy.

E.　Enzyme Studies

III.　CHILD NEGLECT

A.　General considerations

1.　Definition

a.　Neglect is the failure of the parent or caretaker to provide a child under 18 with basic needs such as food, clothing, shelter, medical care, educational opportunities, protection and supervision.

B.　Incidence and Prevalence

1.　Over 1 million cases of confirmed child neglect in U.S. each year.

2.　It is estimated that the incidence of child neglect may be 5 times greater than that of physical abuse.

C.　Medical Considerations

1.　Physical indicators

a.　Failure-to-thrive: height and weight significantly below the fifth percentile for age.

b.　Inappropriate clothing for weather

          c.   Poor hygiene including lice.

          d.   Child abandoned or left with inadequate supervision.

          e.   Untreated illnesses or injuries.

          f.   Lack of safe, warm, sanitary shelter.

          g.   Lack of medical and dental care.

    2.   Behavioral Indicators

          a.   Child is lethargic.

          b.   Begs or steals food.

          c.   Poor school attendance or tardiness.

          d.   Chronic hunger.

          e.   Dull, apathetic appearance.

          f.   Running away from home.

          g.   Reports no caretaker in home.

          h.   Assumes adult responsibility.

D.   Failure-to-thrive

    1.   Definition

          a.   Child shows a marked retardation or cessation of growth. On growth, the child may fall below the third percentile or show no growth over time.

          b.   Failure-to-thrive may result from a medical condition or environmental factors such as neglect, poor parenting skills, or a combination of medical and environmental factors.

          c.   Failure-to-thrive generally presents in children in less than two years of age. Diagnosis is confirmed by admission to hospital and observation for growth when appropriate caloric needs are met.

IV.   PSYCHOLOGICAL MALTREATMENT

A.   General Considerations

    1.   Definition

          a.   Lack of a parent or caretaker to provide a child with appropriate support, attention and affection.

    2.   Psychological abuse is a chronic pattern of behavior such as belittling, humiliating and ridiculing a child. NOTE: Both types of maltreatment may result in impaired psychological growth and development of the child.

B.   Incidence/Prevalence

    1.   Is largely unknown.

    2.   It was thought that all abused children suffered some sort of form of psychological maltreatment as it is the court component of all forms of abuse.

C.   Medical Considerations

    1.   Physical indicators

          a.   Disorders

          b.   Sleeping disturbances

c. Inappropriate bedwetting or soiling
d. Speech disorders
e. Failure-to-thrive
f. Developmental lags

2. Behavioral indicators
   a. Habit disorders such as biting, rocking, head banging, thumb sucking, poor peer relationships.
   b. Behavioral extremes including aggressive vs. withdrawn; sad appearance, apathy, lack of responsiveness, self-destructive behavior, chronic academic underachievement, irrational and persistent fears or hatreds.

Elias Srouji
Kendall Stanford
Roger Thompson

CHRONICALLY RECURRING PROBLEMS IN AMBULATORY PEDIATRICS

Multiple perplexing problems will tend to surface over and over again in the pediatric clinic setting. Many of these visits are simply due to the parent's or child's need to know if they need to worry or not and/or just how much they should worry.

The clinician's role is to sort through the parent's and patient's frustrations and fears to find out what their real concerns are. Attempts should then be made to systematically evaluate whether there is a need for concern. If so, where do we go from here? If not, give parents permission to quit worrying or at least decrease their fears. But do not be trapped into diagnosis by becoming fixated on the parent's or patient's perception of the problem.

Remember that all problems do not need to be solved in a single visit. Most of these problems have more than one method of treatment. Some of these problems may never be totally cured.

The following are several of the common perplexing problems that are seen frequently in Ambulatory Pediatrics.

DIURNAL ENURESIS (Daytime Wetting)

Definition: Lack of bladder control during waking hours in a child old enough to maintain bladder control.

Primary Enuresis - untrained after 2 1/2 years in a developmentally normal child

Secondary Enuresis - previously toilet trained, then regresses
A.   usually voids the entire contents of bladder
B.   occasional seepage of a few drops probably normal
C.   occasional wetting during the first two years post training; not abnormal - usually associated with postponement of voiding secondary to playing, etc.

Etiology

A.   Organic Causes (5% of children with daytime wetting)

   1.   #1 cause - urinary tract infections; often associated with frequency and dysuria; females who use bubble bath may develop daytime wetting associated with a distal chemical urethritis
   2.   ectopic ureter - if patient has continual wetness
   3.   neurogenic bladder; often associated with gait disturbance and poor bowel control

4.   lower urinary tract obstruction leads to bladder distension and overflow incontinence; history of straining at urine, dribbling, or small caliber stream suggest this condition

5.   pelvic masses (such as presacral teratoma, hydrocolpos or fecal impaction); pressure on bladder may lead to stress incontinence with running, coughing, or lifting

B.   Physiologic Causes

1.   vaginal reflux - after voiding, urine seeps out of vagina; most common with obese girls

2.   giggle incontinence - detrusor instability (> 90% `female`); bladder spasms leading to abrupt voiding; many have associated nocturnal enuresis

C.   Psychogenic

1.   stress-related; usually between the ages of two and six years; associated with fear or anxiety (e.g., birth of a sibling, loss of a relative, school-related problems) - irregular, infrequent

2.   resistive child; a child greater than two and one-half years who has not responded to toilet training; resistive and negative about using the toilet; most are boys; often associated with a high-pressure approach to toilet training, including severe physical punishment

INCIDENCE

A.   approximately 1% in 7 - 12 year olds
B.   50 - 60% of these have associated nocturnal enuresis

EVALUATION

A.   History: dysuria, frequency, hematuria, continuous dampness vs intermittent flow, previous UTI, precipitating events, use of punishment or lectures, associated nocturnal enuresis or encopresis

B.   Physical Exam

1.   abdominal exam - rule out bladder distension or fecal impaction
2.   genital exam - perianal sensation, anal tone,
3.   lower back for spinal abnormalities; urine stream assessment

C.   Laboratory: urinalysis, urine culture

D.   If positive physical findings or recurrent UTI, refer for urologic consultation

MANAGEMENT
Treat daytime incontinence before nocturnal

A.   urgency incontinence - stream interruption exercises
B.   stress related - sympathy, support; ask for school cooperation in reducing tension
C.   resistive child - discontinue punishment; offer positive reinforcement for success; encourage positive interaction between parent and child

NOCTURNAL ENURESIS

Definition: The involuntary passage of urine during sleep *occurring greater* than one time per month.

INCIDENCE:

30% at age 4
10% at age 6
3% at age 12
1% at age 18

RISK FACTORS:

A.   familial predisposition
B.   males > females; 60% vs 40%
C.   most have small functional bladder capacity
D.   most without emotional problems
C.   organic etiology in 1-2% (most common UTI)
D.   spontaneous cure rate 15% per year

TREATMENT:

A.   motivational counseling (ages 3-6)
B.   child takes active role
C.   reassurance to parents and child
D.   positive reinforcement for dry nights
E.   decrease family friction
F.   decrease fluids three hours prior to bed time and encourage voiding just prior to bed time
G.   follow-up to give reinforcement
H.   bladder exercises (ages 6 - 8)
      1.   bladder stretching
      2.   stream interruption
      3.   increase early morning fluid intake

I.   enuresis alarms (greater than 8 years) to awaken child with first drops (good success rate); set alarm clock to waken child approximately four hours after retiring

K.   Medications (greater than 8 years; use only if other methods have failed)
   1.   Imipramine - tricyclic, not recommended secondary to potentially dangerous side effects
   2.   Antispasmodics - Ditropan
   3.   Antidiuretics - DDAVP

REMEMBER: Relapses and treatment failures are common.

ENCOPRESIS

Definition: Deposition of formed or semiformed stool in the underwear or other abnormal places occurring after the age of four years.

Prevalence: 1 - 3 % of school-aged children; boys much greater frequency than girls (86%)

Development of Encopresis:

A.   intermittent stool retention/constipation
B.   rectum becomes distended
C.   sensory feedback becomes impaired
D.   rectal wall becomes stretched and unable to contract effectively
E.   stools become harder and larger
F.   painful defecation leads to further retention
G.   soft stool and mucus begins to seep around impacted stool
H.   child may pass large caliber stools

Etiologic Considerations:

A.   early colonic inertia
B.   constipation from early life
C.   parental overreaction may aggravate
D.   child may balk at bowel training
E.   incomplete training
F.   critical life events may thwart attempts to develop continence (e.g., illness, birth of sibling; loss of family member, etc.)
G.   the untrained child may continue to soil then retain when faced with social pressures
H.   toilet aversion; toilet phobia
I.   situational toilet avoidance; new environment (school, daycare, etc.); lack of privacy (children avoid defecation; constipation and encopresis follow)
J.   incomplete defecation; partial evacuation results in constipation;
K.   encopresis common in children with attention deficit disorders

L.   psychosocial/stress induced; may be a manifestation of family problems (e.g., marital strife, abuse, neglect)

Other causes of chronic constipation:

A.   Hirschsprung's disease (aganglionic megacolon) 1:25,000
B.   spinal cord lesions
C.   malnutrition
D.   dietary indiscretions (e.g., lack of fiber or overindulgence on cow's milk
E.   disorders of voluntary muscle function (amyotonia congenita, cerebral palsy, infectious polyneuritis)
F.   metabolic - infantile renal acidosis, diabetes insipidus, idiopathic hypercalcemia

EVALUATION:

A.   thorough history
B.   complete physical exam including rectal exam
C.   abdominal x-ray, and barium enema when indicated
D.   laboratory tests only if suspicion of underlying metabolic disorder
E.   rectal biopsy if signs of Hirschsprung's

MANAGEMENT:

Goal is to attain regular bowel habits and restoration of neuromuscular bowel function.

A.   demystify - reassure that many children have this problem and that the child often <u>cannot</u> feel a bowel movement coming on.
B.   catharsis
          1.   clean out procedure; enemas and laxatives
          2.   follow-up x-ray to prove successful clean out (if necessary)
C.   establish regular bowel habits; sit 10 minutes at least two times per day after meals
D.   mineral oil after clean out
E.   consider need for stool softeners
F.   increase dietary fiber
G.   treatment requires long-term commitment; 20% of cases may have recurrence of symptoms; encourage perseverance
H.   enlist school cooperation; permit bathroom visits when needed; private bathroom if necessary

RECURRENT ABDOMINAL PAIN (RAP)

DEFINITION:

"The presence of at least three discrete episodes of debilitating (abdominal) pain occurring over at least a three-month period during the year preceding the clinical examination." (Apley 1975)

INCIDENCE:

10 - 15 percent of school aged children

PERSONALITY PROFILE:

Two categories:

1) Super achievers, verbal, obsessive-compulsive, sensitive, "older than their years," and
2) Average intelligence, but often immature in speech and behavior when compared to more productive sibling

FAMILY HISTORY:

Often many relatives will have a history of conditions such as irritable colon, spastic colitis, anxiety attacks and mental illness. Positive family history of migraines is also common.

DIAGNOSIS:

Organic Considerations:

A. Occult constipation of childhood; colonic distension leads to crampy abdominal pain.
B. Lactase deficiency
C. Malabsorption (including insufficiency and celiac disease)
D. Chronic ingestions (e.g., lead)
E. Medications - salicylates, steroids, and aminophylline; constipating medications such as Ritalin, narcotic cough medications, anticholinergic medications, Dilantin
F. abdominal and inguinal hernias
G. peptic ulcer disease
H. Crohn's disease and ulcerative colitis
I. rheumatic and collagen vascular diseases
J. Henoch-Schonlein purpura
K. hereditary angioneurotic edema
L. parasitic infections (e.g., giardiases or ascariasis) (Pinworms do not induce

pain)

M late complications of trauma or abuse

N. gynecological conditions (endometriosis, PID, hematocolpos, etc.

O. metabolic derangements, hyperlipidemias, diabetes, porphyria, hypothyroidism, hypocalcemia (other stigmata of these conditions should be clinically detectable

P. hematologic disorders, sickle cell, hemolytic anemia, leukemias, lymphoma

Q. neoplasms

R. Idiopathic hypercalcuria

FUNCTIONAL CONSIDERATIONS

Some studies show an increased number of stressful events in families of children with RAP, sometimes a recent traumatic event.

Often associated with school phobia. Stress related to school situations may trigger attacks. Height and weight are unaffected.

ASSESSMENT:

HISTORY

A. careful assessment of the pain, associated symptoms, triggering events etc.

B. past medical history

C. personality

D. school attendance and performance

E. family history

F. review of systems

PHYSICAL EXAM

A. meticulous - both diagnostic and therapeutic

B. include rectal and pelvic

LABORATORY

A. minimum - CBC, sed rate, UA, PPD, stool for blood, ova, and parasites, liver function tests

B. abdominal x-ray

C. further tests as indicated

MANAGEMENT

A. discuss family concerns; assure parents and child that no major illness is evident

B. alter environment as necessary

C. discuss the fact that the emotional state can effect the GI tract

D. keep diary of episodes and related events

E. medicines, laxatives as needed

F. DO NOT feel pressured to make a diagnosis on the first visit

G. give follow-up and positive reinforcement

H. allow time for parent and child separately

I. refer for psychological evaluation in confusing or refractory cases

RECURRENT HEADACHES

I. Incidence and Prevalence:

    A. Nonspecific, Nonrecurrent Headache:

        1. By 7 years, 40%

        2. By 15 years, 75%

    B. Frequent recurring Headaches

        1. Non migraine, 15.7% by age 15 years

        2. Migraine, 5.3% by age 15 years

    C. Male : Female

        1. Under 15 years 5.5 : 4.3

        2. Over 15 years 4.6 : 9

II. Classification: Useful for evaluation

    A. Migraine

        1. Classic

        2. Common

        3. Complicated (with transient neurological signs, basilar artery, acute confusional)

    B. Non Migraine

        1. Tension: often difficult to differentiate from migraine

            (a) with psychopathology, (b) without psychopathology

        2. Traction: a small percentage, but with serious implications

            a) Intracranial masses

            b) pseudotumor cerebri

        3. Headaches due to diseases of other head and neck structures. e.g. eyes (astigmatism, hyperopia), sinusitis, dental diseases, infections, trauma, or allergy. These are rare causes of recurrent headaches in children.

III. Evaluation:

    A. History: very important

        1. Antecedent events (trauma, loss, stress, etc.)

        2. Onset

    3. Length of history of headaches.

    4. Course of frequency and intensity.

    5. Frequency of of episodes.

    6. Intensity and character of pain episodes

    7. Duration of episodes.

    8. Location of pain.

    9. Presence of warning symptoms (aura)

    10. Associated symptoms and signs.

    11. Time of day of start of episodes.

    12. Does it require cessation of activity?

    13. any aggrevating factors (positional, etc.)

    14. Any alleviating factors.

    15. Family history of headaches.

    16. Psychosocial history.

B. Physical Examination:

    1. Complete examination including blood pressure, skin for neruofibromatosis, phascomatosis

    2. Full neurological examination.

    3. Eye examination: visual acuity, visual fields, Fundoscopy.

C. Laboratory: only if indicated.

D. Imaging: If indicated, MRI is the optimal.

IV.   Traction or Brain Tumor Headaches:

A. Differentiating Characteristics:

    1. Progressive course.

    2. Occurs early mornings.

    3. Position affects intensity.

    4. Vomiting.

    5. Ocular and or neurologic sings must be carefully looked for.

B. Follow Up,

    1. When headache is of less then 6 months history, and no symptoms or signs suggestive of traction haeadches, patient to be seen at frequent intervals (monthly at least) and reevaluated.

    2. Otherwise, appropriate imaging: MRI or CT with contrast to be done.

    3. Imaging to be done in any child less than 4 years old with recurrent or persistent
headaches.

V. Migraine:

    A. Criteria for diagnosis: (Scandinavian)

        1. Periodic, recurrent with free intervals.

        2. Plus any two of the following:

            a) Aura

            b) Nausea

            c) Vomiting

            d) Positive family history.

B. Prognosis:
    1. Better than adults: 10-12% remit per year.
    2. Migraine starting beyond puberty may stay on.
C. Treatment:
    1. Non Medicinal therapies:
        a) Food avoidance?
        b) Biofeedback , Hypnosis, Relaxation.
    2. Medicinal:
        a) Treatment of episode:
            (i) Aspirin or Acetaminophen (most commonly used)
            (ii) Ergotamine: not recommended under 12 years, and even then not more than once a month.
            (iii) An antiemetic such as dimenhydrinate is the mainstay of therapy when vomiting is a major symptom.
        (b) Prophyalctic treatment: indicated only if migraine attacks are frequent or compromise child's achievements.
            (i) Beta-adrenergic blockers e.g. Propranolol. MAKE sure the patient is not asthmatic.
            (ii) Cyproheptadine.

INFANTILE COLIC

DEFINITION:

Paroxysm of irritability, fussing, or crying lasting a total of three hours a day and occurring on more than three days in any one week in an infant less than three months of age.

INCIDENCE

Approximately 10% of infants age one to three months; usually resolves spontaneously by three to four months

POSSIBLE ETIOLOGIES

    A. intrinsic problems - temperamental predisposition, low sensory threshold
    B. extrinsic problems - overstimulating environment, maternal anxiety
    C. feeding problems - underfed/overfed, excessive air swallowed, inadequate burping, milk allergy

DIAGNOSIS

Diagnosis of exclusion:

A. rule out organic causes for excessive crying

B. include detailed history, narrative of the infant's typical day, occurrence and progression of symptoms

PHYSICAL EXAM

A. thorough exam to rule out evidence of organic pathology
B. laboratory seldom indicated

TREATMENT

A. counseling of parents
    1. reassure that infant is healthy
    2. empathize
    3. discuss parental anxiety and psychosocial stressors
B. observe parental handling of infant and intervene appropriately (e.g., decrease overstimulation)
C. discuss the option of <u>not</u> always picking up child if crying occurs when child is dry and well fed
D. medication - controversial, not recommended (Phenobarbital, Bentyl)
E. close follow-up and reassurance

FAILURE TO THRIVE (FTT)

DEFINITION:

A term used to describe infants or young children whose weights are persistently below the third percentile for age on standardized growth charts.

EPIDEMIOLOGY:

3% to 5% of infants under one year of age admitted to the hospital; 70% to 80% of these from non-organic etiology

ETIOLOGY:

A. Non-Organic (most common)

1. inadequate intake the most common final determinant
2. underlying psychosocial issues may play a large part (psychologic stress can inhibit growth hormone production)
3. emotional deprivation and/or physical abuse or neglect may be involved
4. environmental disruption

B. Organic

1. CNS abnormalities
2. malabsorption
3. cystic fibrosis
4. partial cleft palate
5. congenital heart disease
6. endocrine disorders
7. idiopathic hypercalcemia
8. Turner Syndrome and other chromosomal abnormalities
9. renal disease
10. chronic infection
11. rheumatic disorders
12. malignancies

DIAGNOSIS AND EVALUATION:

A. Thorough physical exam

1. look for signs or symptoms of organic pathology
2. careful assessment of height, weight, and FOC
3. observe for signs of physical and emotional deprivation (e.g., apathy, poor hygiene, intense eye contact, withdrawing behavior)

B. Developmental assessment

C. Thorough history
    1. family history; growth patterns of siblings, etc.; history of organic disease in close family members
    2. detailed history of feeding practices and diet
    3. close observation of interactions between parents and child
    4. detailed growth chart
        a. has growth been steady although below the third percentile?
        b. was growth normal and suddenly slowed? If so, at what point?

D. Laboratory

    1. baseline CBC and UA
    2. further tests as indicated by physical signs and symptoms

E. Period of observation in hospital

TREATMENT:

A. address medical problems
B. if inadequate intake, ensure adequate calories for maintenance and catch up growth
C. frequent weight checks
D. indications for hospitalization: severe malnutrition or dehydration, failure of outpatient management, evidence of abuse or neglect, extreme parental anxiety

ATTENTION DEFICIT DISORDER (ADD)

DEFINITION:

Children with short attention span, high distractibility and an inability to ignore extraneous stimuli when trying to attend to a task. They are often impulsive and have difficulty regulating their actions to conform with social norms. They are often hyperactive and have poor frustration tolerance.

CLINICAL MANIFESTATION:

A. as in the definition above
B. emotional and behavioral difficulties common
C. often socially ostracized
D. poor self esteem
E. increased incidence of learning disabilities
F. often reported to be more active than normal from birth on

DIAGNOSIS:

A. thorough history including performance and teacher's perception of the child
B. thorough physical exam including vision, hearing, and neurologic exams (patient may not display their characteristic behavior in the physician's office)
C. children with ADD may show increased numbers of "soft" neurologic signs (e.g., mixed hand preference, impaired balance, astereognosis, dysdiadochokinesia, and problems in fine motor coordination)
D. laboratory not generally helpful
E. behavior rating scales - Conners Parent Rating Scale, Conners Teacher Rating Scale to be sent with parents and teacher for rating over a several day period
F. consider referral for psychometric testing when learning difficulties are present

TREATMENT:

A. counseling; helping parents' understand the child's problems
B. behavior modification - parent and child
C. encourage a structured environment
D. medication - stimulants: Methylphenidate (Ritalin); Dextroamphetamine (Dexedrine); Pemoline (Cylert)
    1. give a clinical trial to reassess with behavior rating scales
    2. use only in conjunction with counseling and behavior modification
E. consider psychotherapy when signs of severe depression or serious affective disturbances are detected

RECURRENT INFECTIONS

DEFINITION:

Infections occuring with a frequency greater than the norm or caused by an unusual or opportunistic organism.

No person escapes their childhood without occasional illness. When does it become necessary to evalulate a child for the possibility of an immune deficiency?

As with most medical encounters, the History and Physical Exam will play the largest role in determining whether a child's infections falls within normal limits or whether futher work-up is desirable. Even with a comprehensive H&P it can at times be difficult to decide; all of the following commonly occur in normal childhood:

Bacterial Infections
> Meningitis
> Acute Otitis Media (multiple organisms)
> Pharyngitis
> Sinusitis
> Pneumonia (unless recurrent or caused by unusual organisms)
> Gastroenteritis
> Cellulitis
> Impetigo
> Urinary Tract Infections

Viral Infections
> Upper Respiratory Infections (colds)
> Lower Respiratory Infections/Bronchiolitis
> Gastroenteritis
> Viral Syndromes/exanthems

Fungal Infections
> Superficial fungal infections
> Thrush

Any of the above can occur in completely immunocompent children, and are not a manifestation of an underlying disorder. Underlying immunodeficiencies can arise from defects in the B cells, the T cells, phagocytic defects, or complement defects. If pursuit of an immunodeficiency diagnosis is warrented, the following is reasonable, in addition to an initial CBC, appropriate X-rays, bone scans, cultures and erythrocyte sedimentation rate:

Quantitative immunoglobulin levels: IgG, IgM, IgA; IgG subclasses
Isohemagglutinin titer to meaure IgM function
Delayed hypersensitivity skin tests for Candida, tetanus toxoid, tuberculin,
> mumps to measure T cell function

function
IgE level
Total hemolytic complement (CH50) to measure complement activity
C3, C4 levels to measure major complement pathway components

Richard A. Wright

I. Introduction.

A. Why Ethics in Pediatric Care?

1. **Ethics is always present** in medical practice. It cannot be avoided because ethics occurs whenever people interact; since the practice of medicine is the occasion for human interaction, ethics is a foundation of medical practices.

2. **History and tradition are keys to understanding** the ethical viewpoints of a society. The values history of a society informs current situations and their analysis. The profession of medicine is also a society whose members are the physicians, whose links are the practices of the profession, and whose values are those of the individual professionals <u>as well as</u> the community of members. Ethics and ethical values are part of this history.

3. **Ethics affects all patient care**, not just hospital care, or intensive care, or end-of-life care. Most ethical issues, in fact, arise in normal patient care situations in the office as well as the hospital or long term care. Some pediatric care responsibilities which regularly raise ethical problems are the following:

   a. Maintaining the **confidentiality** of information.

   b. **Truth-telling** in the information giving process.

   c. Assuring **informed consent**/refusal for treatment.

   d. **Goal setting** during clinical management

   e. Recognizing and dealing with **preferences and values** when making treatment decisions.

4. **Technology always has an impact on ethics** because it changes what can be done. Each new potential for action is an occasion for considering the ethical implications of that action. The more a change effects key aspects of human life, (e.g., ability to earn a livelihood, quality of life, quality of environment, etc.) the more important the ethical considerations. Questioning whether or not new technology should be utilized, is always important, but especially in end-of-life cases.

5. **Ethics is necessary in clinical care** because ethical values always play a role in the decision process. Paying attention to the ethical dimensions of medicine also focuses attention on caring for a person as an individual, not solely as a dysfunctional organ system or disease process.

6. **Ethics enhances patient care** by enabling the physician to make better decisions by considering a greater number of relevant factors. In pediatrics three specific results are noticeable:

a. The best interests of the patient take primacy

b. Family values become recognized in decisions, instead of being hidden.

c. A positive decisions environment is created thus enhancing cooperation and communication.

B. What is Ethics in Pediatric Care?

1. **Ethics is a process which attempts to answer the question, "All things considered, what is the morally right thing to do?"** The problem, of course, is determining what is right. The study of ethics helps with that problem by making clear what general components of "rightness" specific actions need to contain. In addition, knowledge of ethics includes understanding the rational process of ethical thinking, thus making possible an improvement in the process by which right actions are determined (or questionable actions are evaluated).

2. **Ethics is a process of systematic decision-making** which requires accounting for values and value judgments, in a non-neutral way. It is systematic, because, as with all decision making, there are important components which need to be included if there is to be hope of success.

3. **Ethical thinking goes beyond personal beliefs** and deals with the beliefs of others in the decision situation.

4. **Ethical thinking is rooted in a substantial knowledge base** of literature in philosophy and theology, as well as medicine.

5. **The practice of medicine includes the process of ethics**, because medicine involves interpersonal relationships which have basic human values as their foundation. It is therefore impossible to function as a physician and not be engaged in the process of ethics. The important question is how to best accomplish the ethics based reasoning necessary to practice competently.

II. Key Concepts

A. **Basic Principles of Action**. All decisions utilize principles, i,e. basic rules which are accepted by most people, regardless of their socialization. General ethical decision making has four principles which are primary to health care. Although simultaneous application of all four may be contradictory in a specific case, an effort is made to honor the spirit of each principle, and the letter of those which directly affect the situation.

1. **Beneficence** - produce as much good as possible from any action. This does not imply a simple absence of non-good (e.g., harm) but a conscious attempt to cause a positive good. Medicine traditionally recognizes several specific expressions of this principle:

a. **Preserve life**. There are two ethical problems with this expression. First, does it mean always preserving any functioning biology, such that cessation of treatment is never justified? Second, when there is a question about the value of an individual life, for example, the anencephalic infant, the comatose terminal cancer patient, etc., how are treatment decisions to be made?

b. **Relieve suffering**. The absence of pain and discomfort is generally seen as a primary good in anyone's life. The ethical problem is balancing this against other principles. For example, relief of pain which requires life-threatening doses of medication, or palliative surgery which leaves the patient dysfunctional.

c. **Promote the Patient's Best Interest**. The "best interest" of a patient is a frequently stated aim of medical care. "Best interest" is usually determined in part by what is "medically appropriate" but may also be influenced by the patient's prognosis, the parent's wishes for care, social policies, etc.

d. **Improve the Patient's Quality of Life**. The ethical problem is determining how and upon whose values quality of life is determined. Quality of life is essentially determined only by the persons whose life quality is at issue. If that person cannot express that determination, quality of life decisions may be inappropriate.

2. **Nonmaleficence** - avoid harmful actions as much as possible. This principle does not require production of specific goods; rather, it requires a conscious attempt to prevent the occurrence of harm, or, if harm cannot be prevented, minimizing harm. The tradition of health care recognizes three specific expressions of this principle:

a. Prevent Suffering. Situations or actions which may cause suffering should be avoided. If such situations cannot be avoided, every effort should be made to minimize the suffering, with the overall aim being its alleviation as soon as possible.

b. **Prevent Harm**. Situations or actions which may cause harm should be avoided. If such situations cannot be avoided, every effort should be made to minimize the harm, with the overall aim being alleviation of the harmful elements as soon as possible.

c. **Prevent deterioration in quality of life**. Actions which diminish a person's quality of life as they perceive it should be avoided. This necessitates an understanding of the person's views, instead of an imposition of the physician's personal quality of life assessment.

d. **Assure competent, diligent care**. One of the primary causes of maleficence in medicine is unskilled, incompetent or sloppy care. Iatrogenic illnesses are not all accidental or beyond control, nor is blatantly incompetent care.

3. **Autonomy** - competent individuals may determine for themselves the course of their own lives. Although a fundamental right, autonomy is not an absolute, to be honored above all else, without question. Rather, its application is contingent upon at least three factors:

a. **Competence** of the decision maker is a necessary precondition for the exercise of autonomy. Absent competence, a proxy decision maker is required.

b. **Authenticity** determines how the decision fits the norm of an individual's system of values and beliefs. Unlike competence, authenticity is not always necessary, but it lends support to a decision if present, or indicates a potential problem if absent.

    c. **Acceptability** of a decision, like authenticity, is not absolutely necessary, but it lends support to a decision if present, or indicates a potential problem if absent. Disagreement about the acceptability of a decision is a frequent source of ethical conflict in medical practice, especially decisions for non-treatment.

    4. **Justice** - honor the fundamental equality of persons. Although often seen only as a legal principle, justice is first and foremost an ethical principle. For without the ethical basis of justice, rooted in the principle of autonomy, the legal framework for assuring justice would be illogical. Health care issues of justice appear primarily in connection with questions about the allocation of resources and access to health care. An action is usually considered just if it adheres to three guidelines:

    a. Does the action recognize a relevant **equality** of persons?

    b. Is each person treated **fairly**?

    c. Has there been a reasonable attempt to **address basic needs** of the affected persons?

III. **The Decision Process.** Every decision, by definition, is a rational process. Ethical decisions, like clinical decisions, are thus rational processes. The key to effectively handling problems in pediatric care is to recognize the role and importance of ethical factors in the decision situation. Also important is the understanding of how rational process considerations apply to ethical decisions, since many people mistakenly believe that ethics is totally irrational. The key to properly understanding ethics and the role of ethics in decision making, is to see ethics as one of the basic components in any decision process.

    A. **Decision factors** give a decision its content. While there can be any number of different items used in a decision, five basic categories of items heavily factor clinical decision making. These factors link clinical decision making with ethical decision making, because all are present to some degree in every decision situation; importantly, each decision situation can be primarily affected by any of the factors.

    1. **Data** form a basis for all decisions. Although no ethical decision is a function solely of the data, no ethical decision can be made in the absence of data. It is important to recognize the various categories of data which are important, such as medical, social, psychological, etc.

    2. **Action constraints** either prevent or force a specific action. A realistic decision process thus incorporates the relevant constraints placed upon the decision makers in that situation, otherwise the decision is idealistic and usually unworkable. The principles of Beneficence, Nonmaleficence, Autonomy, and Justice often constrain action. Things such as time, personal or social values, personnel or equipment availability, individual skills, etc., also constrain action.

    3. **Values** underlie all human action. The key role of values in the decision process makes it crucial to recognize and understand the value components of a decision situation, for both the patient and the physician.

a. **The roles for values in decision making** include:

(1) **Framing the way things are seen**. Perception is rooted partially in data and partially in interpretation. People learn to see (interpret) situations as congruent with their own value system. Two people can then disagree over whether something is a problem or not, despite a sharing of data.

(2) **Pre-establishing a range of alternatives**. Values predispose a person to accept or reject alternative potential actions in any situation. Alternatives which fit one's value system will be "available" while those which counter that value system will be "off limits."

(3) **Influencing or directing the choice of action**. Just as values predispose a person to accept or reject actions, those values also directly influence the final selection of an alternative for action. In general, a person will not select an "off limits" action.

b. **Value Types** need to be recognized before their importance in a decision situation can be recognized. Each person utilizes many different specific values, but individual value systems generally contain the following types of values:

(1) **Economic values** determine the relative merit of competing claims against economic resources. For example, persons on fixed income may have to choose between paying doctor bills and paying rent.

(2) **Social values** guide interpersonal relationships and establish a framework for professional practice within a community. Racial bias and willingness to do community service are examples of such values.

(3) **Religious values** determine a person's religious viewpoint. Atheism is as much a set of religious values as Judaism or Catholicism. Many religious value systems impose restrictions on medical care which may influence patient decision making. Examples are the Jehovah's Witness refusal of blood products, and Church of the First Born refusing all medical care of any sort.

(4) **Legal values** are not the laws themselves but a person's attitude toward the law and its influence on professional life. Most important is whether the law is seen as an ultimate value (dictating all action) or a subservient value (adjudicating disputes).

(5) **Moral values** are personal beliefs which guide specific actions. These values, such as a belief that nutrition and hydration may never be withdrawn because to do so is murder, are the basis for decisions about what is right and wrong in specific situations where the belief applies.

(6) **Professional values** are imposed upon and accepted by a person who accepts membership in the profession. The appropriateness of these values is determined by the profession as a community, and they may change over time. The anti-surgery injunction of the

Hippocratic Oath and the anti-abortion stance of the early code of the American Medical Association are examples of such values.

4. **Decision theory** is the structural, logical component all medical decisions have by virtue of their process. Four aspects of decision structure are quite important to the ethics process:

   a. **Identify who ought to be the decision maker**. For example, a baby's parent is usually the decision maker. However, with a teen-aged mother who cannot understand her baby's condition, the grandparent may be the appropriate decision maker.

   b. Identify what decision components need to be considered. Not everything is equally important, and not everything needs to be decided at one time.

   c. **Determine how (via what process) the decision should be made**. If, for example, a parent and an adolescent disagree over treatment, should the parent's wishes be automatically followed? Should a court order be sought to declare the adolescent competent for self-determination?

   d. **Facilitate the decision process**. This includes trying to accommodate parental schedules in setting up appointments, being sure the location of the meeting is not intimidating, focusing on parental information needs, etc.

5. **Ethical focus** is the general framework of individual ethical decisions. Even though every person has a unique set of specific values and beliefs, the ethics process focuses on the commonalities inherent in perceived differences between individual viewpoints. Thus, no matter what set of beliefs an individual holds, almost <u>all</u> ethical decisions focus in one of three ways; the key to understanding another person's decision is to determine which of the three is the ethical focus for that person.

   a. **Consequences**.

      (1) **Act to produce the greatest good with the least harm**. The "good" is estimated for each possible action, and the one selected for implementation will be the one intended to produce the best outcome. Estimation of outcome is always relative to the individual situation, but may depend upon prior experience. The variation from case to case arises from different assessments of possibilities for the case in question.

      (2) **Pragmatic considerations** usually affect the decision process. The consequences focus requires **weighing risks and benefits**, goods and harms, according to an identified set of values which define "good" and "benefit." These are then balanced against other things such as institutional rules or professional duties, according to some scheme of relative values or "weights" for individual considerations. Disagreements most frequently arise when different people value or "weigh" things differently.

   b. **Duties**.

      (1) **Act in accordance with the obligations** determined by sets of rules, values, or

professional norms. **Primary duties** are those which have their basis in human nature, while **secondary duties** are based upon human actions. The duty to preserve life is an example of a primary duty, while the duty to renew an expired driver's license is a secondary duty.

(2)   **Duties vary**, but all participants in a decision situation have duties which apply to them. The question is what role those duties play in the final decision.

    (a)   **Professional duties** are imposed by the medical profession through its code of ethics, and by the community which empowers the professional practice. Many duties are distinctive to physicians and require that physicians act in ways which are required of no one else in society. In addition, physicians are subject to the basic duties which apply to anyone who is a professional, e.g., honesty, candor, diligence, competence, integrity, etc.

    (b)   **Care recipients and their proxies** have duties, both to themselves and to others. Self-care, honest communication, collaboration in the decision process, and diligence in accomplishing the collaborative decision, are examples of their duties.

    (c)   **Ancillary duties** accrue to others with a **legitimate** role in the decision situation, e.g., family members, courts, society, and insurance companies. The problem is that these others often try to play an **illegitimate** role, inappropriately talking over or interfering. A frequent ethical problem in medicine is determining who has a legitimate obligation to participate in the decision.

(3) **Pragmatic considerations** rarely influence a decision which is based on duties. The only relevant "weighing" occurs when two different obligations seem to be in conflict and both cannot be achieved.

c. **Rights**.

   <u>(1)</u>   **Act to uphold moral rights** which accrue to individuals by virtue of either their status as persons or societal award. <u>Primary rights</u> are those which have their basis in one's status as a human being, while <u>secondary rights</u> are awarded to people through social actions. The rights to life, autonomy, and privacy are examples of primary rights, while the right to Medicare payments is a secondary right.

   (2)   **Rights vary**, but all participants in a decision situation have rights which apply to them.

    (a)   Professional rights are given to physicians by society and the medical profession, through the regulations and traditions governing the profession. Physicians also have rights which derive from the fact that each physician is a person. Those rights which are distinctive to physicians may require that physicians act in ways which would not be required of others. Beyond that, physicians as persons have the same rights as anyone else.

(b) **Care recipients** have rights which derive from their status as persons, such as the right of autonomy, or the right to protection from harm. They also have rights given by society or specific social entities, e.g., the legal right to informed consent, or rights to care as specified in the American Hospital Association's Patient's Bill of Rights.

(c) **Ancillary rights** accrue to others with a legitimate role in the decision situation, e.g., family members, courts, society, and insurance companies. The problem is that these others often claim, or try to exercise, rights which they do not have. A frequent ethical problem in medicine is determining what rights are legitimate influences in the decision process.

(3) **Pragmatic considerations** rarely influence a decision which is based on rights. The only relevant "weighing" occurs when two different rights seem to be in conflict and both cannot be honored.

B. Decision Procedure

1. Identify the problem

No problem can be resolved until it is first appropriately identified. This requires not only an understanding of the decision factors, but also identification of those factors which are instrumental to the problem.

a. Distinguish problems from issues

Everything which is an issue is not always a problem. For example, confidentiality and privacy are at stake (issues) in any interpersonal interaction. They only become problematic when their violation seems necessary.

b. Distinguish conflicts from dilemmas

A conflict is the inability of individuals to deal with differing viewpoints, value systems, etc. A dilemma is a situation in which there appears to be a need to select from among unsatisfactory actions. The most serious dilemmas arise when facing a decision which seems to require choosing among alternatives which each require a violation of basic moral principles.

2. Identify alternatives for action

No problem can be resolved until some means for its resolution has been identified. Rational problem solving requires identification of alternatives for resolution, so that a decision among alternatives can be made. To attack a problem with only a single-minded approach is to use irrational dogmatism instead of rational problem solving.

a. Identify a wide range of alternatives

The key failure in rational decision making is to overlook appropriate alternatives. The usual way this happens is to identify only two alternatives for a situation, namely "Do it" or "Don't do it." Instead, alternatives should be identified for different ways of "doing it" and different ways for "not doing it."

b. **Identify other people's alternatives**

Identify alternatives that others would consider reasonable, even if you do not. This allows for fuller consideration of the options.

3. **Select alternatives for action**

Once a set of alternatives has been established, it is necessary to select one of those alternatives for action. The selection of the alternatives for action is our answer to the ethical question (I.B.1) "What, all things considered, is the morally correct thing to do?"

4. **Justification**

This is the set of reasons which can be given for the selected alternatives for action. Merely stating one's opinion is not sufficient, since opinions alone have no value. The requirement of rational decision making is that a person be able to explain why they chose the alternative that was chosen. What reasons can be given for the choice? Why was it the appropriate choice? Why were other choices not selected?

5. **Reflection**

After the resolution to a problem as been accomplished, reflection is the activity of reviewing and analyzing the action, as well as the process which led to that action. Reflection is the key to improved decision making in the future. It is the recognition that, despite our best efforts, we can be mistaken. The point of determining this, however, is not blame but improvement for the next similar situation.

IV. **Common Ethical Concerns in Pediatric Care**.

A. **Privacy and confidentiality** affect all aspects of the physician-patient relationship. Based upon recognized patient rights of privacy, respect, and autonomy—the physician has duties to maintain confidentiality. The consequences of not doing so, loss of trust, poorer quality of care, and potential lawsuits—are substantial. The physician's duty to the patient is often challenged by third parties (family, government, insurance companies, employers) who believe they should have access to patient information. The physician, as gatekeeper of patient information, must make a decision whether or not to release information based on ethical considerations of patient's rights.

B. **Truth Telling** is a key component in both the exchange of information and the consent process. Without information which is complete and accurate, a person cannot exercise the right of autonomy, since adequate decision making requires adequate information. When deciding what information to give, the physician must recognize the professional duties of honesty and candor. The consequences of not doing so would include loss of trust and inadequate consent. The physician must then balance the principle of beneficence against the principle of autonomy in judging how and what information to give patients, parents or other decision makers.

C. **Informed consent** is both an ethical and a legal requirement, although the legal clearly has its roots in the ethical right to autonomy. Obtaining consent in pediatric care is just as important as in any other care setting, but often far more complex.

　1.　**Proxy consent** is the norm. Inpatient often encompasses a number of family members in the process. Normal consent process still requires paying attention to the details of the consent process, to assure that a competent person is giving adequately informed consent for treatment modalities that are understood and appreciated.

　2.　Consent is **based upon the best interests of the child** under care, not the proxy decision maker. As guardian of the patient's well being, the physician is morally responsible for assuring such a consent process.

　3.　**State laws** often do not permit parents to refuse medical treatment for their child. In cases of parental refusal, especially involving life-sustaining treatment, consent may need to be obtained through legal means.

　4.　**Adolescents, mature minors, and emancipated minors**, are increasingly recognized to have at least a right to <u>assent</u>, if not outright consent. If a parent consents (authorizing the action), but a child refuses to assent (allow the action) legal resolution may be the only alternative.

　5.　**Children who are wards of the state** fall under consent processes which are encumbered by bureaucratic and legal restrictions.

D. **Goal Setting** in pediatrics care is a combined physician-parent function which depends upon all of the concerns discussed in previous sections. There is an additional role for physician preferences and physician autonomy. Since autonomy is a function of persons, not professions, the physician has autonomy which is as important as patient or parent autonomy. Goal setting allows not only the development of a plan of action for the patient's care, but also articulation of physician values which may influence achievement of that plan. From the ethical perspective, goal setting is the personal level of interaction which focuses attention on the value system which underlies patient care. This permits the involved parties to assess their relationship, as well as the values that direct that relationship.

E. **Parental Preferences and Values** are primary determinants of what can actually be accomplished in a pediatric care setting, regardless of whether inpatient or outpatient. Outpatient settings, however, increase the need for preference and value determination, since implementation of the treatment modality is totally under parental control. Failure to determine patient preferences and values, or work with them in the therapeutic relationship, will increase the risk of non-compliance, thus failure of the treatment regimen. Ethical dilemmas often arise when parent preferences and values conflict with physician judgment concerning appropriate treatment options. Careful attention to parent preferences and values helps to decrease such problems.

V. Clinical Assessment for Problem Identification and Resolution.

A. **Problem Components** are those elements of a decision situation which cause or contribute to ethical problems in pediatric practice. The first step in dealing with ethics in practice is to recognize these components and avoid their pitfalls.

1. **Competence determination** is a necessary component of ethics based decision making. The ethical principle of autonomy assumes that adults are competent but children are not. The burden of proof thus lies on the physician to show that the parent is <u>not</u> competent or that the child <u>is</u> competent. To accept a decision by an incompetent person is ethically as bad as not accepting the decision of a competent person. The physician treating children thus needs to develop competence determination skills to as part of the decision process.

2. **Context** has a powerful role in decision making. If a person is placed in a setting which is frightening, intimidating, etc., their decisions cannot be unaffected. The physician has a responsibility to establish a context of care which diminishes as much as possible these negative influences on the decision process.

3. **Coercion and manipulation** of decisions is not ethically acceptable; persuasion, however, may be required in some situations. The difference between the two is that persuasion attempts, through a good faith interaction and neutral agenda, to inform a person's decision. The aim of persuasion is to present information which allows a person to undergo a change of beliefs and come to agreement with another, e.g., the physician. Coercion and manipulation attempt, through deception, intimidation and misinformation, to affect the outcome, with no attempt to change beliefs. A person who is persuaded to take an action does so from a new belief that the action is correct. A person who is coerced or manipulated into taking an action still believes that the action is incorrect, but is doing it anyhow because of the coercive force.

4. **Understanding** is the key to ethical decision making. A person must understand the information upon which his or her decision is based. <u>Misunderstanding</u> can occur because there is a lack of information, or because the information given is not understood. The two primary causes of misunderstanding are <u>language which is too technical</u> and <u>barriers to understanding</u> such as fear, denial, poor education, etc.

B. **Problem Identification Questions** are interrogatories which assist with the recognition of an ethical problem, or focus a recognized problem into an understandable category for resolution. Whenever there is an affirmative answer to a question, that issue must be dealt with as part of the problem resolution.

1. **Are there specific problems easily identified?** Violations of privacy, breaches of confidentiality, untruthful information, inappropriate utilization of quality of life judgments, inappropriate levels of care, poor consent processes, etc., may be specifically identified as a problem by someone

involved in the situation.

2. **Are there values which conflict?** For example, the parents cannot afford the recommended treatment; religious beliefs prohibit the treatment offered; or the patient prefers quality of life over extension of life.

3. **Are there aspects of the case which do not seem to depend upon medical information?** If all the necessary medical facts are known, but a question about care still remains, the missing elements are most likely value elements. A values history might then be necessary to complete the assessment.

4. **Is there non-technical disagreement over care?** For example, if there is agreement that the diagnosis and treatment are correct, but the patient or parent is still refusing treatment, that is a value issue, not a medical issue.

   a. **Is there patient/physician or parent/physician disagreement?** What is the source of disagreement? Is there an appropriate attitude toward care? Have values been expressed which conflict with the physician's values?

   b. **Is there family/patient or family/physician disagreement?** Does the family have a legitimate and appropriate role in the decision? Does the family interaction help, hinder or threaten care? Is the family seeking its own best interests instead of the patient's best interests?

   c. **Is there disagreement among physicians, or among physicians and other staff?** If so, is it technical disagreement, such as concern with a recommended procedure's effectiveness; or, is the disagreement about such things as the patient's role in care decision, family role, informed consent, quality of life, discontinuing care, etc.?

5. **How has the decision making process been accomplished?** Are the decisions primarily by one person? Is the physician inappropriately trying to control the situation? Is the patient inappropriately trying to control the situation? Has there been appropriate consultation with all those having a legitimate role in the decision?

6. **Are there uncomfortable choices to be made?** Does it appear that no choice of action is really a good one? Does it appear that it might be impossible to do what a consensus would label as 'right'?

VI. Summary

Every physician is engaged in ethics during all aspects of patient care and management. Some cases, such as indigent care, transplantation, HIV infected patients, child abuse, removal of life-sustaining treatment, etc., are especially troubling because they present such complex problems. The process of ethics can be **learned**, however, and **applied** to everyday cases, thereby enhancing our ability to deal with the very difficult ones. Doing ethics is a habit of mind which translates into better medical decisions, thus better patient care.

TEST QUESTIONS

Single Best Answer

1. The best <u>initial</u> laboratory evaluation of an anemic child is

    (A) serum iron determination
    (B) reticulocyte count
    (C) red cell indices
    (D) stool guaiac test
    (E) bone marrow evaluation

2. A two year old male child presents to the pediatircian's office with generalized edema. Examination of the urine shows 4+ protein. A lowered serum protein and albumin and an elevated serum cholesterol level are also present. His blood pressure is normal and no erythrocytes are present in his urinalysis. The definifitive treatment for this disorder is:

    (A) dietary sodium and fluid restriction
    (B) Deitary sodium restriction
    (C) Prednisone
    (D) Lasix
    (E) A renal biopsy followed by intravenous Lasix

3. A 3-year-old boy who was toilet-trained at 18 months begins to wet himself during the day and night. This may be due to any of the following EXCEPT

    (A) diabetes mellitus
    (B) a urinary tract infection
    (C) the arrival of a new sibling
    (D) divorce in the family
    (E) orthostatic proteinuria

4. Of the following, the most likely cause for an acute febrile illness, seen chiefly in the summer and characterized by small vesicles and ulcers surrounded by erythema in the soft palate and anterior tonsillar pillars is

(A)   herpetic stomatitis
(B)   coxsackievirus group A
(C)   streptococcal pharyngitis
(D)   Vincent's stomatitis
(E)   agranulocytic angina

5.   A 3-year-old boy has fever, cough, and a sore throat. He has slightly red conjunctivae and moderate erythema of the soft palate and pharynx. Tonsils are reddened and covered with exudate. The anterior cervical lymph nodes are moderately enlarged. Chest is clear. Leukocyte count is 12,000/mm^3 with 60% polymorphonuclear neutrophils, 2% band forms, and 38% lymphocytes.

Of the following, the organism <u>LEAST</u> likely to cause this infection is

(A)   <u>Hemophilus influenzae</u>
(B)   adenovirus
(C)   beta-hemolytic streptococcus, group A
(D)   <u>Corynebacterium diphtheriae</u>
(E)   Epstein-Barr virus

6.   At a routine visit of a 2-year-old boy, you notice a moderate degree of pretibial bruising. The findings on the remainder of the physical examination are normal.

Of the following, the most appropriate management at this time is to

(A)   order x-ray studies of the long bones
(B)   order determination of the bleeding and clotting times
(C)   request a psychosocial consultation
(D)   suggest limited activity for several days
(E)   reassure the mother

7.   A seven year old boy presents to his physician's office with abdominal pain, vomiting and coke-colored urine. Physical examination reveals a blood pressure of 150/104, and non-pitting edema is present. The boy had been treated by his physician earlier in the month for impetigo. The most important diagnostic studies to determine the etiology of this condition are:
(A)   serum electrolytes
(B)   urinalysis and chest x-ray
(C)   ASO titer and C'3 complement
(D)   EBV titere
(E)   CT scan of the abdomen

8. A 12-year-old boy is referred to you because of pain and swelling below his right knee. He is active in sports, particularly basketball and skiing. On physical examination, there is point tenderness over the anterior tubercle of his right knee.

The most likely diagnosis is

(A) patellar dislocation
(B) osteochondritis dissecans
(C) tear of the collateral ligament
(D) Osgood-Schlatter disease
(E) tear of the medial meniscus

9. Which of the following physical findings in boys is the earliest indicator that puberty has begun?

(A) increasing prostate size
(B) appearance of upper lip hair
(C) increasing penile size
(D) increasing testicular size
(E) appearance of pubic hair

10. An 8-year-old boy became febrile and anorectic four days ago, five days after return from a summer camping trip. Yesterday, a red macular rash appeared on his ankles and wrists. The rash rapidly spread to the entire body, including scalp, palms, and soles, and became more purple and papular. There are now many petechiae and the child complains of headache, malaise, and myalgia.

The most likely diagnosis is

(A) Rocky Mountain spotted fever
(B) anaphylactoid (Henoch-Schoenlein) purpura
(C) meningococcemia
(D) Lyme disease
(E) Kawasaki disease (mucocutaneous lymph node syndrome)

11. The mother of a 2-year-old child with normal growth and appearance is concerned that her child's speech seems delayed. Motor development has progressed normally.

Of the following, the most appropriate next step is to

(A) reassure the mother that her child will likely "catch up"
(B) defer psychometric evaluation until just prior to entry into kindergarten
(C) refer the child for speech evaluation
(D) order computed tomography (CT) scan of the head
(E) perform a standardized developmental screening test (e.g., Denver Developmental Screening Test)

12. Bilateral otitis media develops in a 9-month-old boy. Cefaclor (Ceclor) therapy is begun. Forty-eight hours later, he has a temperature of 39.5 C and has a toxic appearance. He does not interact well with the examiner.

Of the following, the most appropriate next step in management of this infant is to

(A) begin ampicillin, intravenously
(B) begin trimethoprim with sulfamethoxazole, orally
(C) begin chloramphenicol, orally
(D) perform an examination of the cerebrospinal fluid
(E) perform bilateral myringotomies

13. Congenital dislocation of the hip

(A) is common in infants who have a club food deformity
(B) is more likely to occur in girls who are born by breech rather than by cephalic presentation
(C) is not likely to be present if results of physical examination are normal at birth
(D) is best diagnosed by x-ray study of the hips in the first three days of life
(E) is more common in boys than in girls

14. Most full-term infants will regain their birth weight by:

(A) 48 hours
(B) 4 days
(C) 10 days
(D) 30 days

15. What is the expected fluid requirement of a 25 kg child?

    (A)   2,500 cc/d
    (B)   2,100 cc/d
    (C)   1,600 cc/d
    (D)   1,750 cc/d

16. A 5-year-old boy has a sore throat, a temperature of 39^0C (102.2^0F), and enlarged anterior cervical nodes. His fluid intake has been good, and he has not been vomiting. On examination of the posterior pharynx, you find that his tonsils are erythematous and swollen, without exudate.

Your differential diagnosis includes both streptococcal and viral pharyngitis. The diagnostic criterion MOST helpful in distinguishing between these two entities is*

    (A)   presence of exudate
    (B)   lymphadenopathy
    (C)   toxic appearance of the patient
    (D)   headache
    (E)   throat culture

17. Assume you are most suspicious of streptococcal pharyngitis. Your FIRST step is to

    (A)   administer benzathine penicillin intramuscularly
    (B)   obtain a screening test for streptococcal infection
    (C)   start a 10-day course of oral administration of penicillin
    (D)   not treat because the infection is self-limited

18. In a patient who has completed a course of treatment for streptococcal pharyngitis and is asymptomatic, the MOST appropriate management is to

    (A)   culture the family members
    (B)   refer for tonsillectomy
    (C)   perform periodic urinalyses
    (D)   assume the patient is cured

19. Organisms prevalent in the etiology of <u>otitis externa</u> include each of the following <u>EXCEPT</u>:

   (A)   Hemophilus influenzae
   (B)   Pseudomonas aeruginosa
   (C)   Proteus mirabilis
   (D)   Staphylococcus epidermidis
   (E)   Candida albicans

20. A 2-year-old male develops a sudden fever which rises to 106^0F and persists for 3 days. The temperature then abruptly drops to normal and the next day a generalized skin rash appears which lasts for only 18 hours. The most likely diagnosis in this case is:

   (A)   Measles (Rubeola)
   (B)   Chicken pox (Varicella)
   (C)   Rocky Mountain Spotted Fever
   (D)   Roseola infantum (Exanthem Subitum)
   (E)   German measles (Rubella)

21. Of the following signs, which one is <u>not</u> characteristic of scarlet fever?

   (A)   vesicular rash early in course
   (B)   sandpaper rash
   (C)   sore throat
   (D)   strawberry tongue
   (E)   patient may appear quite ill

22. An infant presents to clinic with complaint of straining at stooling. Today mother noticed red blood in the stool today. The most likely cause

   (A)   anal fissure
   (B)   hemorrhoid
   (C)   Meckel diverticulum
   (D)   intussusception

23. Appropriate therapy for group A streptococcal pharyngitis

   (A)   oral penicillin for 10 days
   (B)   Cefaclor (Ceclor) for 5 days
   (C)   Trimethoprim - Sulfamethoxazole (Bactrim) for 10 days
   (D)   all of the above
   (E)   none of the above

24. A 4-month-old boy is seen in the clinic for a WCC. On exam he is well-appearing. It is his first visit to the doctor. You are planning to immunize him. Which immunization would you order

   (A)   DPT   OPV
   (B)   DPT   IPV
   (C)   DPT   OPV   HIB
   (D)   DPT   OPV   MMR

25. You are attending the delivery of a newborn infant. At one minute of life the infant has a heart rate of 60, no respiratory effort, is cyanotic, has poor tone and doesn't respond to suctioning. The infants apgar is

   (A)   0
   (B)   1
   (C)   2
   (D)   3

26. At 5 minutes of life the same infant has been bagged with O_2 and given Narcan, now his heart rate is 120, he is breathing on his own with a strong cry and grimace at suctioning. He is fully flexed. His apgar is

   (A)   8
   (B)   9
   (C)   7
   (D)   unable to determine from information

27. A right parietal cephalhematoma obscures which suture line?

   (A)   none
   (B)   it depends on the size of the hematoma
   (C)   sagittal

28. A 6-week-old infant has had an indolent conjunctivitis since birth and a cough for two weeks with progressive tachycardia and recent dyspnea. Diffuse rales are present, although the infant is not in severe distress. His temperature is 37.8 C (100.8 F). A chest roentgenogram reveals chest infiltrates bilaterally.

The most likely cause of this infant's condition is

(A) bronchiolitis due to respiratory syncytial virus
(B) pertussis
(C) pneumonitis due to <u>Chlamydia trachomatis</u>
(D) pneumonitis due to <u>Pneumocystis carinii</u>
(E) pneumonitis due to group B hemolytic streptococci

29. The infant above should be treated with: (Pick the single best answer)

(A) PO erythromycin for 2 weeks
(B) Na Sulamyd eye drops
(C) PO erythromycin for 7 days
(D) PO bactrim for 10 days

30. The most commonly fractured bone in a difficult delivery is

(A) humerus
(B) clavicle
(C) rib
(D) ulna

31. Which of the following medicines can be given down the endotracheal tube during a resuscitation

(A) Epinephrine
(B) Nicotine
(C) Bicarbonate
(D) Calcium Gluconate

32.	A newborn infant is markedly pale following a crash C-section for abruptio placenta. You are going to give a fluid bolus followed by blood. The most readily available IV access is

(A)	umbilical vein
(B)	umbilical artery
(C)	peripheral IV
(D)	saphenous cutdown

33.	A 15-month-old child has a rectal temperature of 40.5^{0}C, but does not appear to be seriously ill. No specific findings are evident on the physical examination. White blood cell count is 24,000/mm^3. A blood culture is obtained and is reported to be positive. The most likely etiology of the bacteremia is:

(A)	Haemophilus influenzae, type b
(B)	Streptococcus pneumoniae
(C)	Meningococcus
(D)	Staphylococcus aureus
(E)	Streptococcus pyogenes

34.	The mother of a 15-year-old girl reports that her daughter has been complaining for several weeks of intermittent abdominal pain. After the initial examination indicates no abnormalities, which of the following is the most appropriate next course of action?

(A)	ask the mother if her daughter has been having sexual intercourse
(B)	interview the patient alone
(C)	arrange for the patient to receive a prescription for a prostaglandin inhibitor
(D)	schedule an intravenous pyelogram and voiding cystourethrogram
(E)	order a clean-catch urine specimen and culture

True or False

35.	Blood pressure measurements should become part of the routine examination starting at 10 years of age.

36.	There is an increased incidence of purulent otitis media in children with cleft palate.

37.	Hypertrophic pyloric stenosis commonly occurs after 6 months of age.

38.	Urinary tract infection in children is more common in boys than in girls.

39. Infantile "colic" usually occurs in infants under 3 months of age.

40. The full term infant will generally double the birth weight by 5 months of age.

41. Painless rectal bleeding is a common sign in children with Meckel diverticulum.

42. Acute cervical lymphadenitis in children is commonly due to Staphylococcus aureus or group A beta hemolytic streptococci.

43. Circumcision should be performed in boys with hypospadias to prevent recurrent urinary tract infections.

44. Cromolyn is not useful in the treatment of asthma.

45. The most common cause of epistaxis in children is trauma with an underlying bleeding disorder.

46. Oral moniliasis is uncommon in neonates and a diagnosis of congenital HIV infection should be considered.

47. A cephalhematoma can be large enough to cause hyperbilirubinemia when the blood begins to break down.

48. Bronchiolitis occurs most commonly in the adolesecent age group.

49. The pulmonary vascular markings on chest x-ray in pulmonary stenosis are markedly increased.

50. Aortic stenosis produces a holosystolic murmur.

Answers to Test Questions

1. C	26. D
2. C	27. A
3. E	28. C
4. B	29. A
5. A	30. B
6. E	31. A
7. C	32. A
8. D	33. B
9. D	34. B
10. A	35. F
11. C	36. T
12. D	37. F
13. B	38. F
14. C	39. T
15. C	40. T
16. E	41. T
17. B	42. T
18. D	43. F
19. A	44. F
20. D	45. F
21. A	46. F
22. A	47. F
23. A	48. F
24. C	49. F
25. C	50. F